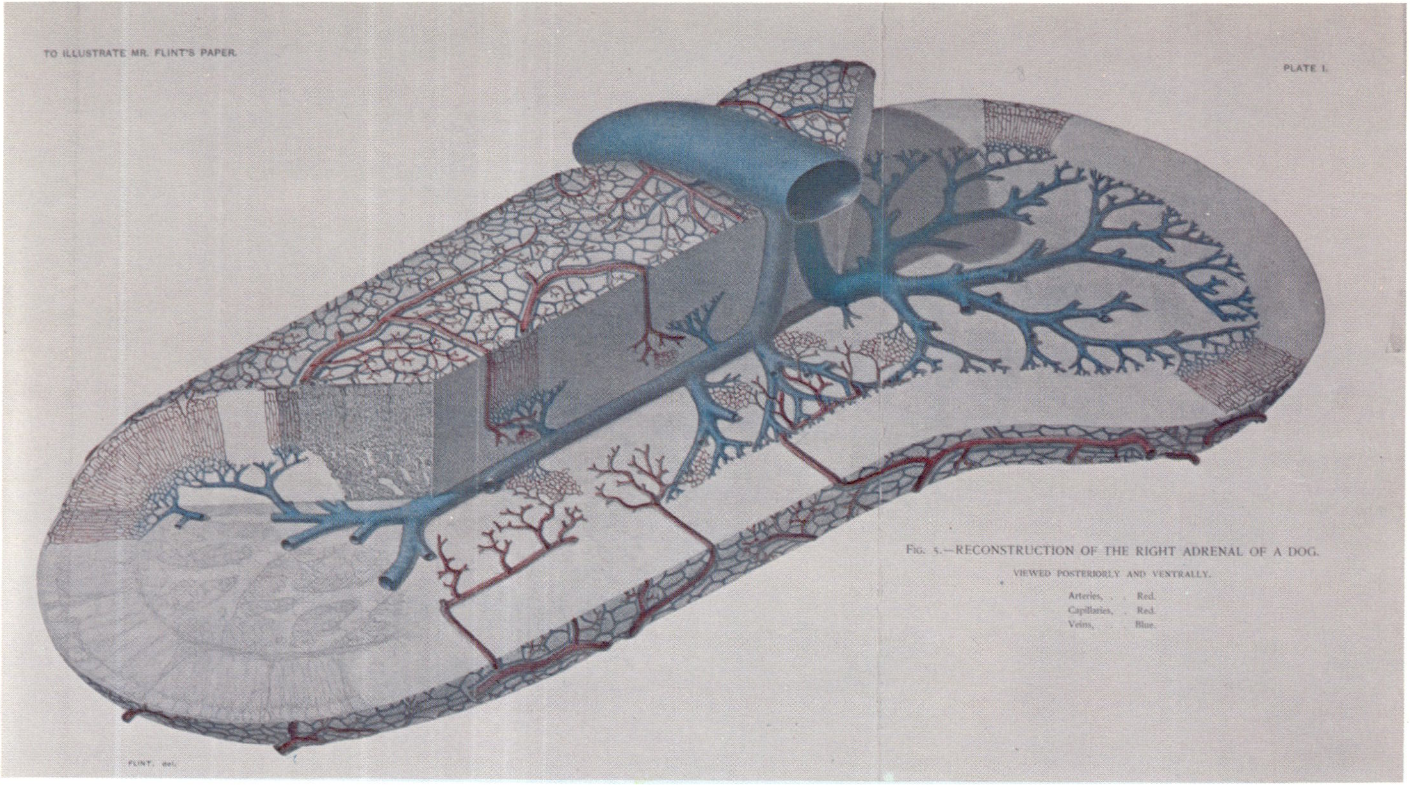

Reconstruction of the circulation of the right adrenal gland of the dog, by Joseph Marshall Flint in 1900. Flint was a fourth year medical student when this work was published. He was the first to appreciate the adrenal portal venous system. This system perfuses the adrenal medulla with blood high in adrenal cortical hormone content. (By courtesy of the Johns Hopkins University Press.)

Surgical Disorders of the Adrenal Gland: Physiologic Background and Treatment

Modern Surgical Monographs

Series Consultant

Richard H. Egdahl, M.D.
Professor of Surgery
Boston University School of Medicine

Surgical Disorders of the Adrenal Gland:

Physiologic Background and Treatment

Timothy S. Harrison, M.D.
Professor of Surgery
University of Michigan Medical School
Ann Arbor, Michigan

Donald S. Gann, M.D.
Professor of Surgery
Director, Department of Emergency Medicine
Professor, Biomedical Engineering
The Johns Hopkins University School of Medicine

Anthony John Edis, M.D.
Consultant, Section of Surgery
Mayo Clinic
Rochester, Minnesota

Richard H. Egdahl, M.D.
Professor of Surgery
Boston University School of Medicine
Boston, Massachusetts

GRUNE & STRATTON
A Subsidiary of Harcourt Brace Jovanovich, Publishers
New York San Francisco London

Library of Congress Cataloging in Publication Data
Main entry under title:

Surgical disorders of the adrenal gland.

Includes bibliographies.
1. Adrenal glands—Diseases. 2. Adrenal glands —Surgery. I. Harrison, Timothy S.
[DNLM: 1. Adrenal glands—Surgery. WK790 S961]
RD599.S94 617′.461 75-6963
ISBN 0-8089-0864-2

Grune & Stratton, Inc.
111 Fifth Avenue
New York, New York 10003

Library of Congress Catalog Card Number 75-6963
International Standard Book Number 0-8089-0864-2
Printed in the United States of America

Contents

Foreword

Descriptions of the surgical treatment of adrenal disease appear in almost all contemporary surgical texts dealing with general surgery either in its narrow or broad sense. Is it a good idea for still another specialized book to compete for space in the crowded time, awareness, and bookshelves of modern medical students, resident physicians and interested health care professionals in general?

There is no answer that will suit everyone. Each of the authors has, and continues to devote, a major effort to basic research in adrenal physiology. We believe this orientation to fundamental research has benefited patients under our care in a way that nothing else could, and our goal is to emphasize again that basic science and good medicine are not separate entities but part of the responsibility modern physicians feel to their patients.

Facts, as such, are less important to the modern medical student than an awareness of what facts are important, of how to continually inform himself of progress and, above all, how to sense and grasp the inspiration and excitement inherent in studying critically, and trying to understand the lessons both patients and investigative laboratories generate. If any of this spirit comes across in this book, we will consider our efforts to have been rewarded amply.

Numerous acknowledgements should be made. Sabbatical leave from one university has been a help to one of the authors. Continuing investigative support from the National Institutes of Health to each of the authors has permitted research programs to continue.

Our treatment of the history of the adrenal gland was helped immensely by John Blake and Peter Olch of the National Library of Medicine, the staff of the Medical Historical Collection of the Yale University Medical Library, and Ms. Sutton of the Wellcome Foundation Library for the History of Medicine in London. Dr. Elmer Belt of Los Angeles and Professor John Keele of Staines, England have tolerantly given time and interest to several questions, particularly those surrounding Leonardo da Vinci. Both are internationally recognized da Vinci scholars and their insight and knowledge have been particularly helpful. Professor Sergio Damiani, Secretary of the Vatican Archives, kindly searched their material for communications between Pope Julius II and Leonardo da Vinci. Mme. Adriana Salem of Paris and M't. Joli, LeThollenet, Provence was particularly helpful in the considerations involving Professor Henri Mondor. Charles G. Child, 3rd, contributed insight concerning Diemerbroek and two friends and colleagues, René Mornex of Lyons and Glenn Geelhoed of Washington, D.C. have been a stimulus and help in a variety of different ways. An excellent translation of large excerpts from Eustachius' "Opuscula Anatomica" was made by William Klykylo, a medical student with large talents both in medicine and classical studies. Richard Prager, a surgical research fellow, translated the appropriate publications of Brown-Sequard. The original illustrations of Karen Waldo of the Dartmouth–Hitchcock Medical Center and of Denis Lee of the University of Michigan speak for themselves. Figures 4-1 through 4-14 obtained courtesy of the publisher, from stages of art preparation for full color *Manual of Endocrine Surgery,* by AJ Edis, L Ayala, and RH Egdahl, Springer-Verlag, New York, Inc., 1975 (in preparation).

Dr. Luis Ayala of Caracas, Venezuela, was most helpful in providing insight and background for a portion of the chapter on surgical approaches to adrenalectomy.

Numerous colleagues, medical students, research fellows and laboratory co-workers have contributed to the laboratory and clinical work mentioned and continue to ask fundamental questions indispensable to the atmosphere of critical inquiry the authors have tried to maintain investigatively and clinically.

1 April 1975

T.S.H.
D.S.G.
A.J.E.
R.H.E.

1

Historical Perspectives of the Adrenal Gland

"The glands lie upon the kidneys, flattened and elongated as if they were little placentae."

Eustachius, 1563.[4]

Bartholomaeus Eustachius was impatient and dissatisfied with the prevailing scientific dogma of Rome in his day, the mid 16th century. He discovered and was impressed by many inaccuracies in the anatomical "truths" of Galen, daVinci, and Vesalius; rejecting tact, he was bluntly outspoken in his criticism of the existing body of scientific fact. Regarding the adrenal glands Eustachius' sharply worded comments speak eloquently. "I have judged it proper to write at this point concerning certain glands of the kidneys carelessly overlooked by other anatomists. I would have desired that this type of gland not have been overlooked by earlier anatomists and by those who today pursue this art and who have written quite long treatises on the parts of the human body, especially since they represent themselves as factual. They have, in fact, followed the errors of others and have done so so painstakingly as to not uncommonly seem more contentious than interested in anatomical verity."[4] Convictions such as these removed him, one gathers, from accepted scientific circles in Rome.

Eustachius' small "Opuscula Anatomica" published in 1563 contains his first four anatomical plates (Fig. 1-2). This work was given a limited printing and was largely unknown in its day.[5] In fact, these four plates are of the organs of the urinary tract and are remarkably vivid, in part because the sketches were engraved onto copper plates

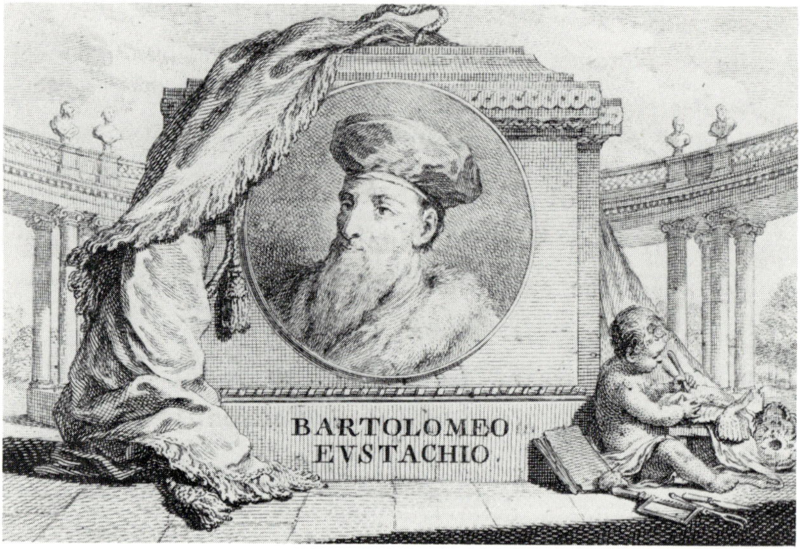

Fig. 1-1. Bartholomaeus Eustachius, 1524–1574. Wood cut from Brombilla, G. A.: Storia della Scoperte Fisico Medico-Anatomico-Chirurgiche, Milan, 1780–1782, 2 volumes, Courtesy of the National Library of Medicine, Bethesda, Maryland.

from which they were reproduced. They are thought to be the first copper plates used for reproduction of anatomical drawings. In the photograph of Eustachius' plate number 1 (Fig. 1-3), one can appreciate his sensitivity for anatomical detail. One also notes the adrenal glands and Eustachius' feeling for their potential importance. So far as can be determined, prior to this description, the adrenal glands had never been appreciated or sketched.

Eustachius continued a life of scientific inquiry using careful anatomical dissection and drawing. He died in 1610, largely unrecognized for his scientific contributions. Almost 200 years later Pope Clement XI discovered the large collection of anatomical plates of Eustachius in the library of the Vatican City and presented them to his physician, Lancisi. Lancisi was impressed by the brilliance, accuracy, vivid detail, and remarkable anatomical insight of the plates, particularly with respect to the dental nerves; with the encouragement of Morgagni, Lancisi published all of the original plates, including the first four of the urinary tract, giving appropriate credit to Eustachius. The "Lancisi" anatomy, was an immediate and overwhelming success. It was subsequently translated into several other languages and went through many editions.

BARTHOLOMAEI

EVSTACHII

SANCTOSEVERINATIS MEDICI
AC PHILOSOPHI
OPVSCVLA ANATOMICA.

Quorum numerum & argumenta auersa pagina indicabit.

Cum Priuilegijs Summi Pont. Illuſtriſſ. Senatus Veneti, Sereniſſ. Francorum Regis, & Catolicæ a Cæſareæ Maieſtatis.

VENETIIS,

M D LXIIII.

Vincentius Luchinus excudebat.

Fig. 1-2. Title Page, "Opuscula Anatomica," 1563, Bartholomaeus Eustachius, Courtesy of the National Library of Medicine, Bethesda, Maryland.

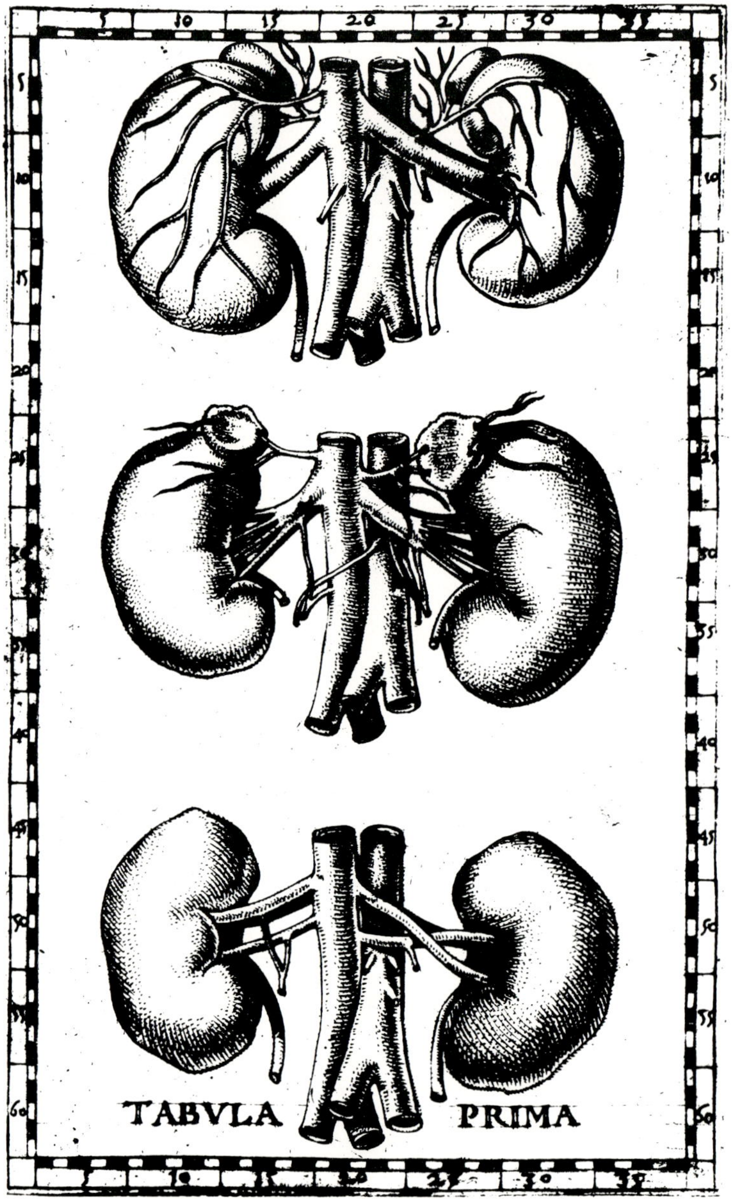

Fig. 1-3. Eustachius' original plate depicting the adrenal glands for the first time. The glands are viewed from the posterior aspect and their differing locations represent extremes of anatomical variations encountered by Eustachius in his dissections. Courtesy of the National Library of Medicine, Bethesda, Maryland.

It is clear that prior to the first Lancisi edition in 1714, the adrenal glands had become recognized through the scientific world and speculation was great as to their function. In 1694, for example, Diemerbroek[3] in a respected and somewhat colorless anatomical text of the day alludes to the "Deputy Kidneys," includes a crude diagram, and refers to the current speculation about the function of the adrenals.

" 'The Capsule Kidneys' by Julius Casser are called the Deputy Kidneys; by Wharton the Glandules adjoyning to the nervous plexure; and by Bartholomaeus, the Capsule Atrabiliary" (Capsules for black bile).

"The use of these glandules is unknown. Spigelius thinks 'em made to fill up the vacuum between the kidneys and the diaphragma. Others think they support the division of the Reteform'd plexure of nerves. Riolanus (thinks) they are of no use to men grown to maturity . . . Glisson believes they separate the juice that serves the nourishment of the nerves from the rest of the blood . . . Wharton believes that there is a certain juice exonerated into these little coffers (glandular spaces) from the plexures of the nerves upon which they lean; which Juice, however, flowing from thence into the veins, may there be useful for other purposes. And, therefore, it is to be hop'd that all practisers, both physicians and anatomists, will for the future observe these parts (adrenal glands) more diligently, and by frequent dissections of dead carkasses inform themselves what diseases their disorder may occasion."

The opinion has been expressed by Girod[6] that Leonardo daVinci described the adrenal glands in 1510, 53 years before the first plates of Eustachius. daVinci allegedly dissected 40 cadavers by special dispensation of Pope Julius II. The plates of these anatomical drawings are said, by Girod, to show clearly the adrenal glands. Girod's assertion can be questioned on several grounds; from da Vinci's notes, it is certain that papal dispensation was not routinely required for human dissection in 16th century Florence. In addition, da Vinci's existing plates' depicting the urinary tract lack any detail that is even vaguely suggestive of the adrenal glands. The Vatican Archives contain no record of a dispensation from Pope Julius II to da Vinci, nor are there any of da Vinci's anatomical drawings in the Vatican Archives. Finally, Henri Mondor,[8] cited by Girod as the source for da Vinci's priority, does not, in fact, more than mention as an uncertain possibility that da Vinci appreciated the existence of the adrenal glands. Professor Mondor, it can be noted, is remembered with affection and respect by his academic friends and colleagues in Paris. Mondor, a Professor of Orthopedic Surgery, was known for his scholarly discernment and extracurricular interests in the arts. In particular, he was recognized as an authority on the works of the French poet Valery.

Sacrificial dissections in the Jewish temples described by Moses in Leviticus 4:9 and 7:4 have, on occasion, been interpreted to allude to the adrenal glands but, as Girod makes clear, Hebrew scholars cannot substantiate this contention.

One leaves the question of priority for the description of the adrenal glands impressed by the uncompromising scientific spirit of Eustachius, skeptical of claims made for da Vinci's priority and struck by the fact that no clear insight into the function of the adrenals was to emerge until roughly 300 years had passed after Eustachius' discoveries.

Thomas Addison, one of the "Great Men of Guys" (hospital in London) flourished professionally in an era when clinical observation provided new insights in medical knowledge. Addison saw, in 1855,[1] two things; one was a series of 11 patients with the same clinical disorder characterized by wasting, weakness, vitiliginous rash, and bronzing of the skin. No treatment was adequate; they all died. His second observation was that in all 11 patients the adrenal glands were destroyed.

In his adrenal monograph,[1] in addition to focusing attention on the specific symptomatology of adrenal insufficiency, Addison was greatly concerned with understanding organ function as displayed by disease. "If pathology be to disease what physiology is to health it appears reasonable that in any . . . organ the laws of the former will be as . . . signficant as those of the latter. Remarkable are the suprarenal capsules, the atrabiliary capsules of Casper Bartholomaeus; it is as a first and feeble step towards an inquiry into the functions . . . of (the adrenals), suggested by pathology, that I now put forth the following pages."[1]

Numerous attempts to understand the function of the adrenal glands followed Addison's monograph.[7] Those of the "erratically brilliant" Brown-Sequard in Paris can be cited as descriptive of difficulties inherent in experimental work of the time.[2]

Brown-Sequard and Trousseau together observed a postmortem exam on a patient who had died from Addison's disease. Brown-Sequard was stimulated by this postmortem exam to study the simple question of whether or not the adrenal glands were necessary for life. A large number of confusing experiments resulted. Bilateral adrenalectomy was performed on 44 rabbits, 5 dogs, 2 adult cats, 9 guinea pigs, and 2 mice. Unilateral adrenalectomy was performed on 16 rabbits, 5 guinea pigs, 2 cats, 2 adult dogs. In comparable species mean survival time was always longer, about 23 hours, in those animals with unilateral adrenalectomy than it was in the animals with total adrenalectomy the mean survival of which tended to be around 10 hours but varied somewhat with the species. The curious thing is that the animals with unilateral adrenalectomy did not survive longer. However, Brown-Sequard does allude to experiments of the "distinguished anatomist M. Gratiolet" who had 2 guinea pigs as long term survivors after unilateral adrenalectomy. Two of Brown-Sequard's later dogs lived 8 days after being ". . . depouille's d'une seule capsule surrenale." One earlier dog would probably have lived longer, Brown-Sequard assures us, if he had not eaten poison by accident.

The significance of Brown-Sequard's experiments was undeniably cloudy but, nevertheless, still appreciated by Trousseau. Brown-Sequard predicted on the basis of these experiments that adrenal integrity would be shown to be necessary for life. It was not long before many others did so.

As acute and chronic adrenal insufficiency became solidly established in physicians' minds, treatment with dried extracts of beef adrenal cortex were used for replacement therapy. As the purity of these extracts improved, their effectiveness increased. Such extracts were in use up until the time of World War II and can scarcely be regarded as "history."

Determination and an incredible amount of hard chemical purification and analysis enabled Edward Kendall of the Mayo Clinic and Thaddeus Reichstein in Switzerland to identify and synthesize hydrocortisone, one active principle among dozens of steroids in adrenal extracts. Next hydrocortisone was demonstrated to be an effective life sustaining agent inadequate in no important way as replacement therapy in patients with classical Addison's disease or adrenal insufficiency from any cause. The remarkable, if transient, therapeutic effect of hydrocortisone in rheumatoid arthritis was soon appreciated by Philip Hench at the Mayo Clinic. Something of the impact of Reichstein, Hench, and Kendall's discoveries on the medical scientific world of the late 1940s can be gathered from their citation in 1950 by the Faculty of Medicine of the Royal Institute of Queen Caroline of Sweden for the Nobel Prize in Physiology and Medicine.[9] The Nobel Committee granted its prize, "for their discoveries relating to the hormones of the adrenal cortex, their structure, and biological effects."[10]

Clearly by 1950 the stage was set for the remarkable scientific advances of the past 25 years. These advances provide deepening insight into the basic and clinical physiology of the adrenal gland and its diseases.

REFERENCES

1. Addison T: *On the constitutional and local effects of disease of the suprarenal capsules,* Samuel Highley, 32 Fleet Street, London, 1855, Reprinted in Facsimile by Dawson's, 16 Pall Mall, London, 1968
2. Brown-Sequard CE: Recherches experimentales sur la physiologie et la pathologie des capsules surrenales, Archs gen Med 2:385, 572, 1856
3. Diemerbroek I de: *The anatomy of human bodies.* W Salmon (trans), Printed by W. Whitwood, Angel and Bible, Little-Britain, 1694
4. Eustachii B: Opuscula Anatomica, Printed by Vincentius Luchinus, Venice, 1563, Excerpts from an Unpublished Translation by William M. Klykylo
5. Garrison FH: *An introduction to the history of medicine,* ed. 4. Philadelphia, W. B. Saunders, Co., 1929 (Reprinted, Dec. 1966).
6. Girod C: *Les surrenales,* in Lecons sur les Glandes Endocrines, Simep, Edit., Lyons, 1968
7. Keele K: Addison on the "supra-renal capsules," an essay review, Medical History, 13:2, 195, 1969
8. Mondor H: *Anatomistes et chiurgiens,* Editions Fragrance, Paris, 1949
9. Nobel Lectures, Physiology or Medicine, 1942–1962, Elsevier Publishing Company, 1964, Amsterdam, London, New York, 837 pages.
10. Sourkes TL: Nobel prize winners in physiology and medicine, 1901–1965, Revised Edition, 1966, Abelard-Schumann, London, New York, Toronto, 464 pages

2
The Adrenal Cortex

PATHOPHYSIOLOGY OF ADRENOCORTICAL DISORDERS

The Zona Glomerulosa

BIOSYNTHESIS OF ALDOSTERONE

Aldosterone is the principal secretory product of the zona glomerulosa, or outer zone of the adrenal cortex. Most of the aldosterone is synthesized by sequential modification of cholesterol taken up from the blood. The principal biosynthetic steps are outlined in Figure 2-1. The side chain of cholesterol is cleaved first to form pregnenolone. This cleavage is controlled by angiotensin II and, to some extent, by ACTH, both of which are presumed to act through the second messenger cyclic adenosine monophosphate (cAMP). The rates of the subsequent biosynthetic steps are affected by the concentrations of appropriate enzymes and the presence of co-factors. One of these is of particular importance at the step at which desoxycorticosterone is converted to corticosterone. This step appears to be highly potassium dependent, and it is generally believed that it is at this site that potassium exerts its principal effect on biosynthesis of aldosterone. There is also some evidence that there is by-product inhibition by 18-hydroxycorticosterone of the conversion of corticosterone to 18-hydroxycorticosterone, and that this inhibition may be indirectly related to the exogenous sodium load.[24] Thus, the

Cholesterol

↓

20α-Hydroxycholesterol

↓

Pregnenolone

↓

Progesterone

↓

11-Desoxycorticosterone (DOC)

↓

Corticosterone

↓

18-Hydroxycorticosterone

↓

Aldosterone

Fig. 2-1. Outlined are the principal biosynthesis steps involved in the formation of Aldosterone.

physiological control of secretion of aldosterone is a direct consequence of the control by external factors of these three critical steps in biosynthesis.

PHYSIOLOGIC CONTROL OF SECRETION OF ALDOSTERONE

Angiotensin. The two principal physiologic stimuli to secretion of aldosterone are a decrease in effective blood volume[2] and an increase in concentration of potassium.[60] In addition, other stimuli to increased secretion of ACTH will also lead to phasic increases in secretion of aldosterone (see below). The influence of diminished effective blood volume accounts for the response of secretion of aldosterone to bleeding, restriction of sodium intake, and assumption of the erect posture. There is a normal circadian rhythm of aldosterone secretion, but this can be abolished entirely if the subject remains in a reclining position throughout the day.[72] In all of these cases, the increased secretion of aldosterone is mediated through increased presentation of angiotensin II to the zona glomerulosa,[23] though this need not be the sole factor leading to increased biosynthesis of aldosterone. Angiotensin II is a peptide formed in blood from an hepatic α-globulin, angiotensinogen. The cleavage of this globulin is controlled by renal release of the enzyme renin. Although the release of renin is probably determined by at least three factors, including renal arterial perfusion pressure, the sympathetic nervous system, and distal tubular delivery of sodium ion,[84] the sympathetic control appears to dominate under most physiologic circumstances, including modest hemorrhage.[52] The relevant sympathetic activity is in turn controlled by the activity of atrial and carotid baroreceptors, whose integrated function serves to measure effective blood volume.[53] The baroreceptor control of release of renin, as well as of release of ACTH (see below) accounts for previous observations of baroreceptor control of secretion of aldosterone.[4]

Following cleavage of angiotensinogen, the decapeptide angiotensin I is formed in blood. Angiotensin is converted to the active octapeptide angiotensin II by the action of a converting enzyme. Although this enzyme is present to some extent in blood, its highest concentration appears to lie in the lung, so that most angiotensin II is formed during the course of passage of angiotensin I through the lung.[74] There is, however, some intrarenal conversion of angiotensin I to angiotensin II. Angiotensin II is removed from blood by the action of an enzyme, angiotensinase. However, changes in the activity of this enzyme do not appear to play a major role in the control of circulating levels of angiotensin II.

The presentation rate of angiotensin II to the adrenal is naturally a function of the rate of adrenal blood flow. Accordingly, it seems reasonable to believe that in shock, when adrenal blood flow is severely limited or abolished, there may be insufficient production of aldosterone. However, at this time, flow dependence of secretory rates of aldosterone has not been demonstrated, but is presumed from a similar demonstration for cortisol.

Potassium. Increases in dietary potassium or in potassium administered by infusion will lead to prompt increases in secretion rate of aldosterone. Conversely, potassium depletion will lead to decreased secretion of aldosterone. It has long been known that potassium ingestion will lead to renal loss of sodium and conversely. However, the effect of potassium on secretion of aldosterone has been shown to be completely independent of changes in sodium balance.[40] As indicated above, the dominant effect of potassium seems to be related to its influence on the biosynthesis of corticosterone from desoxycorticosterone. However, there is some evidence that potassium also acts at an earlier step in biosynthesis as a co-factor in the action of angiotensin II.[58]

The renal excretion of potassium occurs as a result of secretion into the distal tuble and collecting duct under the influence of aldosterone and in exchange for sodium ion. Accordingly, in the presence of high levels of aldosterone, potassium loss or retention becomes a function of the rate of presentation of sodium in the distal nephron. Because of this, potassium may be retained during salt retention and lost during salt loading. The retained or lost potassium will in turn influence the rate of secretion of aldosterone. This rather complicated mode of control becomes important in the differential diagnosis of primary aldosteronism (see below).

ACTH. The acute administration of ACTH or its acute release as a result of a physiologic stimulus, which may range in intensity from loss of blood to the anxiety surrounding the taking of an examination, will lead to an acute increase in secretion of aldosterone. In the normally controlling system, however, the continued administration of ACTH will gradually cease to be effective, as blood volume increases and leads to a reduction in release of renin.[5] However, certain patients have been identified in whom secretion of aldosterone appears to be continuously responsive to normal or slightly elevated release of ACTH. This finding has led to the suggestion that there is an additional mode of control

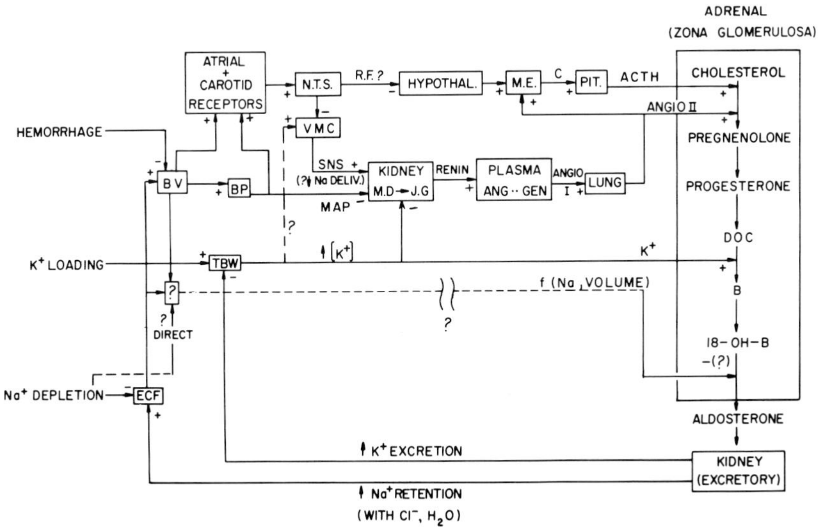

Fig. 2-2. Signal flow in the control of secretion of aldosterone +, stimulation; —, inhibition. RF, reticular formation; C, corticotropin releasing factor; NTS, nucleus tractus solitarius; VMC, vasomotor center; SNS, sympathetic nervous system; BV, blood volume; BP, blood pressure; MAP, mean arterial pressure; Na DELIV., sodium delivery; MD, macula densa; JG, juxtaglomerular apparatus; TBW, total body water; DOC, desoxycorticosterone; B, corticosterone; 18-OH-B, 18-hydroxycorticosterone; ECF, extracellular fluid.

of aldosterone secretion, probably involving inhibition of secretion, which is abnormal in these patients.

Other Modes of Control. The above finding that not all persons with increased concentrations of renin or angiotensin in the blood have increased secretion of aldosterone, and the demonstration in animals that changes in secretion of aldosterone may take place in the absence of kidneys and in the absence of changes in pituitary function or of levels of potassium, have led to the suggestion that there is at least one additional factor involved in the control of secretion of aldosterone.[38] It has been demonstrated both in dogs and in rats that sodium ingestion will inhibit the conversion of corticosterone to aldosterone, possibly by increasing by-product inhibition.[10] This effect cannot be mediated through the renin–angiotensin system or through potassium. Its precise nature remains in doubt, but is an active focus of current studies. Figure 2-2 shows a "block diagram" representation which reflects our current understanding of the control of aldosterone.

OVERPRODUCTION OF ALDOSTERONE

Primary Aldosteronism with Adenoma. Sustained overproduction of aldosterone may result from the presence of adrenocortical adenoma. Under this circumstance the secretion of aldosterone is autonomous in the sense that it does not change in response to changes in presentation of angiotensin II. In fact, during sustained overproduction of aldosterone, the release of renin and thus the formation of angiotensin II is suppressed by the expansion of the blood volume that results from sodium retention. However, because of changes in potassium retention secondary to changes in sodium load, there may be an apparent effect of salt ingestion on secretion of aldosterone, even in this situation. This apparent sodium dependence, which is in fact potassium dependence, has given rise to the term "semi-autonomous."

Sustained hypersecretion of aldosterone may also accompany hyperplasia of the zona glomerulosa, which may take either a nodular or diffuse form. As indicated above, in the diffuse form overproduction appears to be dependent in some way upon the release of ACTH; it may be suppressed by administration of an exogenous steroid such as dexamethasone. In contrast, no etiologic factor has yet been identified in primary aldosteronism with nodular hyperplasia. Plasma levels of renin and of angiotensin II are low, and there is no evidence for dependency on ACTH. This clinical finding has also given rise to search for another factor controlling secretion of aldosterone which may be of clinical importance. However, as indicated above, no such factor has yet been identified.

Whether the pathological factor is an adrenal tumor or hyperplasia the pathophysiological syndrome resulting from excess production of aldosterone is approximately the same. There is increased renal conservation of sodium and thus of water, deriving from a renal tubular action of the hormone. The enhanced sodium conservation leads to expansion of the extracellular fluid volume and, thus, of the blood volume. Because there is no 'sink' into which this fluid can flow, both cardiac preload and afterload are increased, and systemic hypertension results. The expansion of the extracellular fluid volume tends to affect other renal factors which normally control sodium excretion, leading to enhanced delivery of sodium to the distal portions of the nephron. This enhanced sodium delivery in the presence of increased levels of aldosterone leads to increased renal losses of potassium and hydrogen ions. Hypokalemia and alkalosis result. In the presence of persistent hydrogen ion loss, ammonia production is stimulated. Furthermore, because of inhibition of proximal reabsorption of sodium, loss of bicarbonate ion is also accentuated. These factors combine to lead to the production of a persistent alkaline urine, which is characteristic of the syndrome of primary aldosteronism.

Bartter's Syndrome. In some patients renal production of renin is sustained and high, despite adequate sodium ingestion and normal blood volume. Most of these patients are children and it has been suggested that there is an ineffective vascular response to angiotensin II, leading to a sustained stimulus to release of renin.[6] This release leads in turn to increased blood levels of angiotensin II, increased production of aldosterone, and renal wasting of potassium and hydrogen. Children with this syndrome have an accompanying growth failure. The pathogenetic mechanism outlined has not, however, been firmly established.

Renin Producing Tumors. Recently some cases have been described that present a syndrome of renin excess and apparent aldosteronism, secondary to a renal tumor which secretes renin. In this situation, as in the case of Bartter's syndrome, both blood levels of renin and aldosterone will be high at the same time. In the absence of some other basis for the increased renin in the presence of increased aldosterone, the clinician should be led to the suspicion of such a tumor.[15]

Renal Artery Stenosis and Malignant Hypertension. As indicated above, decreased perfusion pressure within the kidney, leading to decreased mean arterial pressure at the juxtoglomerular apparatus in the afferent arteriole, leads directly to increased release of renin. Such a mechanism obtains if there is a partial stenosis of the renal artery resulting from an arteriosclerotic plaque or from fibromuscular hyperplasia or a congenital abnormality or, more rarely, a renal arterial aneurysm. Alternatively, decreased perfusion pressure may result from lesions within the renal arterioles themselves. Such a phenomenon occurs in the presence of malignant hypertension, where there is arteriolosclerosis.[61] In either case, increased release of renin follows with increased production of angiotensin II in the blood. This may lead to an accelerated form of hypertension per se. It will also lead to stimulation of secretion of aldosterone. However, not all patients with renal artery stenosis and increased blood levels of angiotensin II have increased blood levels of aldosterone, suggesting again that there may be an alternative mechanism for inhibition of aldosterone secretion.

Decreased Effective Blood Volume. As indicated above, a decrease in effective blood volume will lead to increased secretion of aldosterone primarily through increased release of renin. Such a circumstance, commonly termed secondary aldosteronism, occurs in clinical states such as hepatic cirrhosis, congestive heart failure, and nephrotic syndrome. The mechanism appears to be the same whether the decrease in effective blood volume results from trapping of blood within the abdomen or from inadequate cardiac action to excite barorceptor activity or from renal loss of albumin leading directly to decreased total plasma volume. In addition, decreased sodium intake and hemorrhage will both lead directly to decreased effective blood volume and, thus, to increased secretion of aldosterone.[61] Such factors contribute to the renal retention of sodium following surgery and trauma.[88] However, it has been shown repeatedly that renal conservation of sodium following trauma and surgery is, to a large extent, independent of adrenal secretion of aldosterone.[39]

UNDERPRODUCTION OF ALDOSTERONE

The production of aldosterone may be below normal in a number of pathological states as well as in several physiological ones. The physiologic conditions leading to underproduction of aldosterone are those associated with salt loading, expansion of the blood volume, or a diet that is deficient in potassium. The mechanism in each of these cases is clear and directly related to our understanding of the control of secretion of aldosterone. The ability to decrease secretion of aldosterone by expansion of the blood volume or by ingestion of salt is useful as a diagnostic tool in the demonstration of autonomous secretion by an adrenal tumor as described below. The underproduction associated with low potassium leads to an apparent 'semi-autonomy' which may produce a diagnostic enigma as described subsequently.

The pathological conditions associated with underproduction of aldosterone include diseases of the adrenal gland involving destruction of the gland as in Addison's disease. Furthermore, deficiency of aldosterone production has been described in association with adrenogenital syndrome in circumstances in which 11- or 21-hydroxylation enzymes are absent.[83] Secretion of aldosterone may also be low in cases of orthostatic hypotension associated with sympathetic insufficiency. Here the defect probably relates to underproduction of renin in response to the stimulus of the erect posture. Finally, it has been shown that approximately 30 percent of hypertensive patients present with subnormal renin.[59] These patients received a great deal of attention initially because it was thought that they might represent a group of patients with primary aldosteronism. However, their production of aldosterone was shown subsequently to be less than normal and their renin secretion was shown not to respond to salt deprivation and maintenance of erect posture. The mechanism involved in this group is not yet clear. Some persons favor the

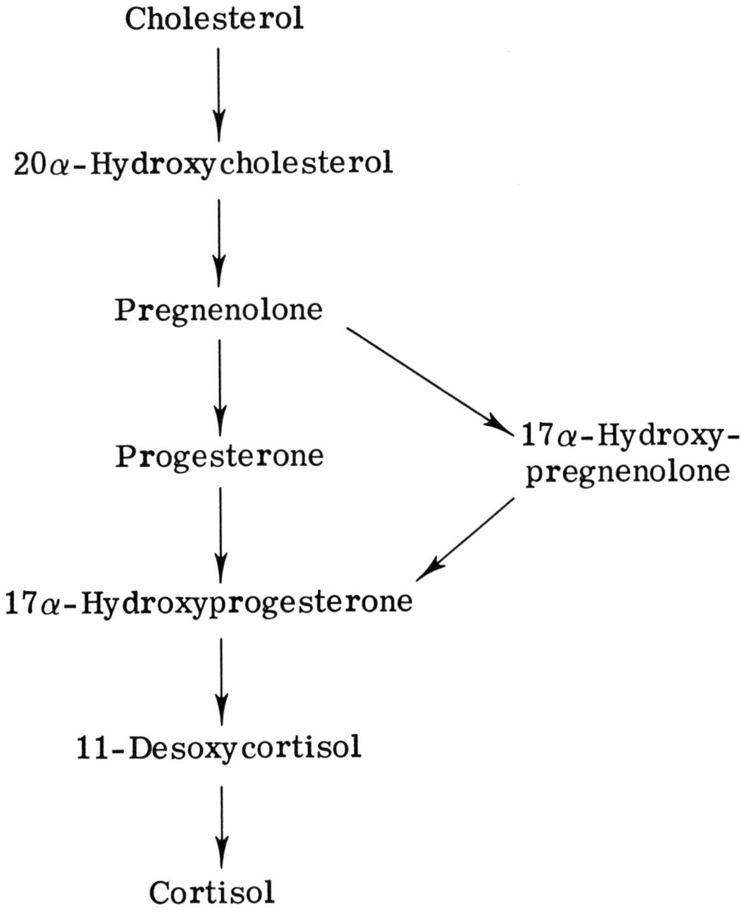

Fig. 2-3. Steps in the biosynthesis of Cortisol from cholesterol are shown.

hypothesis that the underproduction of renin is a direct result of the high blood pressure, whereas others believe that an adrenal steroid may be responsible for this syndrome. Some recent evidence suggests that this steroid may be 18-hydroxydesoxycorticosterone.[69]

The Zona Fasciculata and Zona Reticularis

BIOSYNTHESIS OF CORTISOL

Cortisol is the principal secretory product of the zona fasciculata of the adrenal cortex. Cortisol is synthesized by sequential modification of cholesterol taken up from the blood. The principal biosynthetic steps are outlined in Figure 2-3. The side chain of cholesterol is first cleaved to form pregnenolone. This cleavage is under the control of ACTH, which is thought to act through cyclic adenosine monophosphate. At this point the biosynthetic pathway diverges. Some pregnenolone is reduced directly to progesterone, whereas some is hydroxylated in the 17 position to form 17α-hydroxypregnenolone. The principal biosynthetic pathway then converges with the alternative reaction to form 17-hydroxyprogesterone. This is then converted into 11-dexoxycortisol or compound S by hydroxylation in the 21 position. Finally, hydroxylation in the 11 position converts compound S to cortisol. As in the case of the zona glomerulosa, there is little storage of the final secretory product, so that biosynthesis and secretion are closely coupled. The control of the biosynthetic process takes place in two ways. The principal minute to minute control is exerted by control of the rate of synthesis of pregnenolone, which is in turn a function of the rate of presentation of ACTH. The other biosynthetic steps apparently relate to the availability of the appropriate enzymes. The induction of these enzymes seems also to be a function of ACTH, acting more slowly through control of protein synthesis, which in turn derives from production of mRNA. The failure to induce these enzymes in the absence of ACTH leads to diminished sensitivity of the adrenal cortex to ACTH after hypophysectomy[76] whereas induction of increased amounts of enzyme lead to hypersensitivity to ACTH after sustained presentation of ACTH as in Cushing's syndrome.

PHYSIOLOGICAL CONTROL OF SECRETION OF CORTISOL

As described above, the principal physiologic stimulus to increased secretion of cortisol is increased presentation of ACTH to the adrenal. Increased presentation of ACTH is in turn a function of ACTH concentration in blood and of adrenal blood flow rate. The secretion of cortisol has been shown to be dependent upon this blood flow rate and to be directly correlated with the rate of presentation of ACTH per se.[82] The concentration of ACTH in plasma is directly related to the rate of release of ACTH from the pituitary gland. This rate is in turn controlled by the rate of the presentation to the pituitary of corticotropin releasing factor (CRF) a peptide neurohormone released from the hypothalamic median eminence into the hypophysial portal circulation.[87] The rate of release of CRF can be both stimulated and inhibited by neural signals from other areas of the hypothalamus and from other parts of the central nervous system.[43] In addition, the rate of release of CRF from the median eminence can be influenced by a number of humoral factors. These include cortisol itself, which inhibits the rate of release of CRF.[35] The degree of inhibition is a function both of the level of cortisol presented and of the rate of presentation.[22] This serves as a basis for both level-sensitive and rate-sensitive feedback at the hypothalamic site. Furthermore, the release of CRF can be increased by the presentation of either angiotensin II[32] or of vasopressin[47] to the median eminence. To complicate the picture further, there is some evidence that both of these substances act on the pituitary as well, to inhibit or facilitate the release of ACTH in the presence of constant rates of presentation of CRF.[51,86] The overall physiologic effects however, are always in the same direction.

The level of CRF available for release fluctuates in a circadian rhythm with a dominant peak of release of CRF and thus of ACTH at approximately 6:00 a.m. and a nadir about 12 hours later. In addition to this overall circadian rhythm there is also episodic release of CRF and thus of ACTH and thus of cortisol. This episodic secretion was first identified by Hume, who described "puffs" of ACTH being released into the circulation.[54] It has been shown that episodic secretion of ACTH is necessary to maintain the induction of adrenal enzymes required for the secretion of cortisol. Thus in the absence of such episodic release of ACTH, the adrenal sensitivity to ACTH diminishes and secretion of cortisol is limited. Under normal circumstances, ACTH release occurs approximately every 3 hours[49]. There has, however, been no demonstration whether this is in response to some underlying rhythm or in response to a physiologic stimulus. There is some evidence that carotid baroreceptors are involved in the maintenance of episodic secretion of ACTH.[31]

The release of ACTH is stimulated by a wide variety of physiologic phenomena, which have been grouped together under the term stress. The stimuli include pain, hemorrhage, tissue trauma, general sensation (including sound, touch and light) hypoglycemia, cold, and certain emotional states such as anger and anxiety. There are, in addition, a wide variety of pharmacological stimuli, including ether anesthesia, other anesthetic agents, and histamine.[34,87] The physiologic mechanisms underlying the response to these stimuli have been explored in detail only for the responses to trauma and hemorrhage. In the case of trauma it has been shown that sensory afferent nerves[26] and pathways in the spinal cord[77] are required for mediation of the response. Within the brain stem there appears to be a relatively discrete pathway to the anterior hypothalamus, which leads directly to production of CRF.[41] Many of the synapses of this pathway appear to be cholinergic.[46] In the case of hemorrhage, the decrease in blood volume[37] is sensed primarily by afferent receptors located in the atria and the carotid arteries, which are

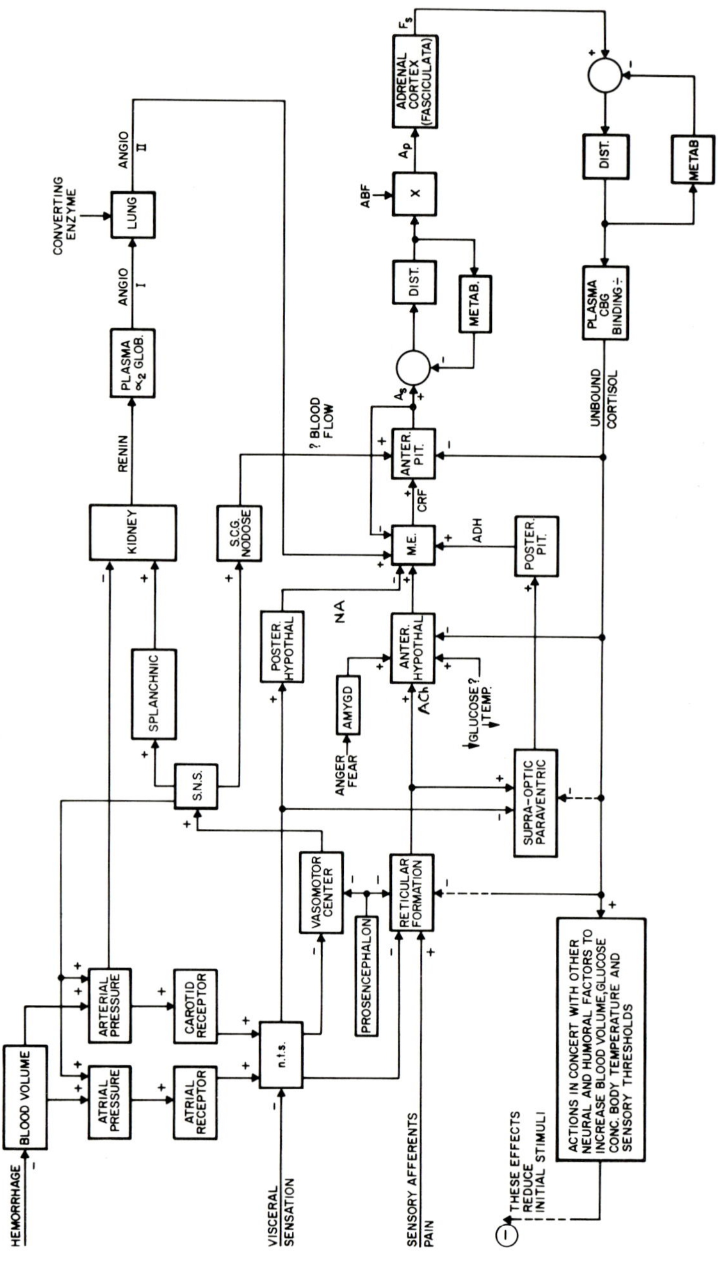

HEMORRHAGE
BLOOD VOLUME
ATRIAL PRESSURE
ARTERIAL PRESSURE
ATRIAL RECEPTOR
CAROTID RECEPTOR
VISCERAL SENSATION
n.t.s.
SENSORY AFFERENTS PAIN
VASOMOTOR CENTER
PROSENCEPHALON
RETICULAR FORMATION
S.N.S.
SPLANCHNIC
KIDNEY
RENIN
PLASMA ∝2 GLOB.
ANGIO I
CONVERTING ENZYME
LUNG
ANGIO II
S.C.G. NODOSE
POSTER. HYPOTHAL
NA
ANGER FEAR
AMYGD
ANTER. HYPOTHAL
ACh
GLUCOSE? TEMP.
SUPRA-OPTIC PARAVENTRIC
POSTER. PIT.
ADH
M.E.
CRF
ANTER. PIT.
? BLOOD FLOW
As
DIST.
METAB.
ABF
X
Ap
ADRENAL CORTEX (FASCICULATA)
Fs
DIST.
METAB
PLASMA CBG BINDING
UNBOUND CORTISOL
ACTIONS IN CONCERT WITH OTHER NEURAL AND HUMORAL FACTORS TO INCREASE BLOOD VOLUME, GLUCOSE CONC. BODY TEMPERATURE AND SENSORY THRESHOLDS
THESE EFFECTS REDUCE INITIAL STIMULI

sensitive to the degree of stretch.[19,31,35,37] Signals reach the brain stem through baroreceptor afferents in the vagus and glossopharyngeal nerves and then pass to the hypothalamus to reach both posterior and anterior sites.[44] The more posterior positions in the hypothalamus appear to be related to tonic inhibition of release of ACTH, whereas the more anterior positions appears to be related to stimulation of release of CRF.[43] There is some evidence that the inhibitory component of this pathway involves noradrenergic synapses.[34] Furthermore, other brain stem structures appear to inhibit the release of CRF. These include sites in the cerebral cortex, septum, and hippocampus. The degree of convergence of these inhibitory components has not been ascertained at present. There is some evidence that there may be a hypothalamic corticotropin inhibitory factor (CIF) as well as CRF. However, whether there is combined stimulation and inhibition of release of CRF, or combined stimulation and inhibition of release of ACTH, or both, there are certainly both stimulatory and inhibitory components of the control system at the cerebral level.[87]

The concentration of cortisol in the blood is a function not only of the rate of secretion of cortisol but also of the rate of destruction of the hormone. The rate of destruction is in turn a function of the degree to which the hormone is bound to a plasma α-globulin, transcortin, as well as to the distribution of cortisol in body fluids. Only the unbound hormone appears to be active and the concentration of unbound hormone must thus be viewed as the resultant action of secretion, distribution, binding and metabolism.[34] The metabolism of cortisol takes place primarily in the liver by the reduction of the A ring of the steroid, but recent evidence indicates that there is a significant degree of destruction of cortisol within the gastrointestinal tract.[63] Cortisol acts on a myriad of metabolic functions throughout the body to produce a wide variety of effects. However, many of these, such as an increase in plasma volume, an increase in blood glucose, and a decrease in sensitivity to sensory stimulation may be viewed as offsetting well-defined stimuli to release of ACTH.[33] In this sense, the metabolic response to the hor-

---

Fig. 2-4. Signal flow in the control of secretion of cortisol. +, stimulation; −, inhibition; SNS, sympathetic nervous system; nts, nucleus tractus solitarius; SCG, superior cervical ganglion; NA, norepinephrine; ACh, acetyl choline; ME, median eminence; ADH, vasopressin; CRF, corticotropin releasing factor; A_s, secreted ACTH; ABF, adrenal blood flow; X, multiplication; A_p, presented ACTH; F_s, secreted cortisol; CBG, cortisol binding globulin; Dist., distribution; Metab., metabolism. (Reprinted, with permission, Ref. 35.)

mone may represent a sort of overall feedback system. Whether this generalization is uniformly applicable remains in doubt, however. In addition, as discussed above, the free cortisol may inhibit release of CRF and of ACTH by actions on the hypothalamus and pituitary to form a negative feedback system. The overall operation of this system and thus of the control of secretion of cortisol is shown in Figure 2-4.

In addition to the diminished sensitivity of the control system as a result of increased levels of cortisol (negative feedback), the portion of the system controlling release of ACTH also responds positively to a stress. Thus one stimulus to secretion of ACTH enhances sensitivity to a second stimulus. This physiologic facilitation has been described only recently[21] but appears to be responsible for the maintenance of the ability of the system to respond to a second stimulus even though peripheral levels of steroids may be increased. Under special circumstances it can be demonstrated in isolation.[21,36]

OVERPRODUCTION OF CORTISOL

Excessive production of cortisol may result primarily from excessive secretion by an adrenal tumor or secondarily from excessive release of ACTH. The latter may stem either from a pituitary tumor or increased release of CRF. As in the case of other tumors, the etiology of an adrenocortical tumor producing cortisol is unknown. However, from the point of view of pathophysiology, the excess of cortisol produced feeds back on hypothalamic and hypophysial sites to reduce plasma levels of ACTH nearly to zero. Such tumors also exhibit very limited sensitivity to ACTH. The diagnosis rests upon these physiologic features, as exhibited by high rates of secretion of cortisol, insensitivity to steroid feedback, and low plasma levels of ACTH.

Adrenocortical hyperplasia with excessive secretion of cortisol may occur in the presence of a pituitary adenoma. Adrenocortical hyperplasia associated with a basophilic adenoma of the pituitary was first described by Cushing.[20] This situation, however, accounts for only about 1 percent of pituitary tumors and is an infrequent cause of adrenal hyperplasia. Chromophobe adenomas of the pituitary are more common.[11] Their occurrence may also be induced following total adrenalectomy for Cushing's syndrome. In this case they may be recognized by a syndrome of hyperpigmentation associated with an enlarging mass in the pituitary region (Nelson's syndrome).[73] The etiology is thought to be associated with excessive presentation of CRF to the anterior pituitary in the absence of steroid feedback.

The most common cause of adrenocortical hyperplasia with excess production of cortisol is excess release of CRF. From the physiologic considerations discussed above, this might occur if there were excessive stimulation of release of CRF as in chronic stress, or failure of the feedback mechanism, the circadian rhythm, or the release of inhibition of CRF release. Adrenocortical hyperplasia has been reported in cases of intense emotional stress.[14,42] Furthermore, absence of circadian rhythm and resistence to steroid feedback are characteristics of this syndrome. The precise mechanisms involved remain unknown. Interestingly, however, episodic secretion of cortisol and thus presumably of CRF and of ACTH persists in Cushing's syndrome with adrenocortical hyperplasia.[49] The diagnosis of adrenocortical hyperplasia rests upon the physiologic mechanisms involved. The demonstration of excessive and bilateral secretion of cortisol in the presence of normal or increased ACTH, but with impaired sensitivity to steroid suppression is of major significance in making the diagnosis. The presence of a pituitary adenoma can be detected physiologically by the demonstration of insensitivity to CRF. Increased physiologic release of CRF may be brought about by blocking the production of cortisol through the use of an antagonist of 11-hydroxylation (metyrapone) usually reflected by increased urinary excretion of 17 hydroxysteroids and by increased plasma content of compound S.

UNDERPRODUCTION OF CORTISOL

Absent or limited secretion of cortisol is associated with primary adrenal failure, enzymatic defects of the biosynthetic process, pituitary failure, and situations in which presentation of ACTH may be limited. Primary adrenal failure, or Addison's disease, may occur directly by an autoimmune process or may be secondary to tuberculosis. The resulting syndrome is the result of absence of cortisol with reversal of its metabolic effects. Thus patients present with hypoglycemia, hyperkalemia, fever, and contracted blood volume and hypotension. There is excess production of ACTH and hyperpigmentation follows.

Syndromes involving deficiencies of most of the hydroxylating enzymes involved in the biosynthesis of cortisol have been described. The most common defect is in the step involving 21-hydroxylation. In this case cortisol cannot be formed and excessive secretion of androgens results. Since these substances cannot inhibit release of ACTH, its production is increased and leads to overproduction of 17-ketosteroids.[1] Some 17-hydroxyprogesterone is converted to preganetriol, the presence of which is diagnostic. In some cases the secretion of aldosterone is also impaired, with resulting salt wasting. However, in most cases the excess secretion of ACTH is sufficient to compensate for the enzymatic block to an extent that permits secretion of adequate amounts of aldosterone.

Adrenocortical insufficiency with diminished secretion of cortisol may be associated with panhypopituitarism. This may be associated with tumors of the pituitary which do not produce ACTH or with pituitary failure secondary to intrapituitary hemorrhage or infarction. In any case, diminished levels of cortisol in the blood are associated with decreased or absent levels of ACTH.

Secretion of cortisol may also be limited in the presence of normal or increased levels of ACTH if adrenal blood flow is limited. This may occur in the presence of adrenal thrombosis, which has been reported following a trauma to the back.[85] It may also occur in shock since adrenal blood flow is severely limited when mean arterial pressure falls below 60 mm Hg.[50] Persistent adrenocortical insufficiency has been observed in some few patients who have recovered from profound shock.

OVERPRODUCTION OF ANDROGENS AND ESTROGENS

As indicated above, sex hormones are produced in excessive amounts in the presence of enzymatic blockades to synthesis of cortisol with resultant increase in ACTH. However, there must be an additional factor controlling the biosynthesis of androgens and estrogens by the adrenal since Mills has shown that the adrenal glands of normal children will not respond even to massive amounts of ACTH with much increase in production of 17-ketosteroids.[70] Furthermore, the inability to reduce estrogen to zero in oophorectomized females with breast cancer treated with corticosteroid suppression also suggests that the production of sex hormones by the adrenal may be under the control of another pituitary factor. The mechanisms remain poorly understood, however. Androgens and estrogens may also be produced in excessive amounts by primary adrenal cortical tumors. They may present as virilizing syndromes in the female or as feminizing syndromes in the male. The diagnosis may be confirmed by appropriate venous catheterization.

PRIMARY ALDOSTERONISM

Diagnosis

Twenty to thirty million people in the United States currently suffer from hypertension. Of these, it has been estimated that at least 200,000 (1–2 percent) are hypertensive on the basis of primary aldosteronism, a potentially curable disorder.[18,65]

There are two main types of primary aldosteronism: (1) aldosterone-producing adenoma (APA), or classical Conn's syndrome; and (2) idiopathic hyperaldosteronism (IHA), which is associated with bilateral adrenocortical hyperplasia.

Sixty-five cases of primary aldosteronism were seen at Boston University Hospital during the 10 years from 1962 to 1972, a solitary adenoma was found in 47 (70 percent) and bilateral hyperplasia in 19 (30 percent). Other rare causes of primary aldosteronism which have been reported include carcinoma of the adrenal cortex, congenital aldosteronism, and glucocorticoid remediable hyperaldosteronism, a form of the disease most often seen in children, in whom treatment with replacement doses of glucocorticoid hormones restores the blood pressure to normal levels and corrects the metabolic abnormalities.

Primary aldosteronism is characterized by an autonomous overproduction of aldosterone which results in sodium retention, potassium depletion, *suppressed* renin activity, and hypertension. It should be distinguished from secondary aldosteronism in which there is *elevated* plasma renin activity (PRA) with overproduction of aldosterone.

Secondary aldosteronism is commonly seen in the various edema states, in which effective blood volume is decreased as a result of the pooling of sodium in the edema reservoir; they include nephrotic syndrome, cirrhosis with ascites, congestive heart failure, and "idiopathic" postural edema. In such cases the renin–angiotensin system operates as a homeostatic mechanism to conserve sodium and to restore diminished effective blood volume. Potassium depletion may result, but secondary hypersecretion of aldosterone does not influence blood pressure. Secondary aldosteronism may complicate renovascular hypertension or the accelerated (malignant) phase of essential hypertension. Treatment with oral contraceptives may also cause secondary aldosteronism; estrogens increase plasma renin substrate levels and can induce such a significant elevation in PRA as to raise the aldosterone secretion rate.

PATIENT RECOGNITION

Unfortunately, the excessive production of aldosterone in primary aldosteronism produces few overt clinical stigmata; unless a high index of clinical suspicion is maintained, the diagnosis may be missed.

The condition affects more women than men, with a peak age incidence in the 30s and 40s. Usually the hypertension is mild; malignant or accelerated hypertension does occur but it is uncommon. More than half the patients have persistent frontal headache, but there is no one feature of the hypertension which can be regarded as distinctive. Conn[16] has emphasized the symptoms of muscle weakness, polydipsia, and nocturnal polyuria which occur as a consequence of the potassium wastage and hypokalemia of aldosterone excess. But some 15 to 20 percent of patients do not exhibit spontaneous hypokalemia and are thus clinically indistinguishable from patients with essential hypertension. It is clear that one cannot rely on clinical features to distinguish those hypertensive patients who have primary aldosteronism from those who do not.

OUT-PATIENT SCREENING OF HYPERTENSIVE PATIENTS FOR ALDOSTERONISM

From a cost-effective standpoint it is not practicable to screen all patients suffering from hypertension by determining aldosterone secretion or excretion rates. Realistically, only selected patients should undergo detailed laboratory study. The criteria for selection, as suggested by Melby,[65] should include: (1) episodic or persistent, spontaneous hypokalemia (serum K^+ <3.5 mEq per liter); (2) hypokalemia occurring shortly after initiation of thiazide diuretic therapy (patients with primary aldosteronism exhibit a marked sensitivity for developing hypokalemia with thiazides); (3) hypokalemia after salt loading.

Salt loading provides a simple and practical means of screening an out-patient hypertensive population for aldosteronism. Sodium chloride is administered in a dose of 2 gm, 3 to 4 times daily for 4 days, in addition to the normal diet. The total salt intake will then approximate 200–240 mEq per day. The serum potassium level is obtained on the morning of the 1st and 5th days; if it falls to the value below 3.5 mEq per liter, aldosteronism should be strongly suspected. The extra salt intake in these patients is like fuel to a fire; in the presence of sustained, autonomous aldosterone secretion, the increased amount of filtered sodium delivered to the distal renal tubule simply serves to feed the aldosterone-dependent sodium–potassium exchange to result in increased kaliuresis. Salt loading in normal subjects, or in hypertensive patients who do not have aldosteronism, invokes a compensatory decrease in aldosterone secretion, the salt load is excreted, and the serum potassium does not change.

Spironolactone Screening Test. Further indirect evidence of sustained, excessive secretion of aldosterone can be obtained in the Out-Patient Clinic by observing the response in blood pressure to treatment with spironolactone. Spironolactone is a competitive antagonist of aldosterone; given in a dose of 400 mg per day, within a few weeks it restores the blood pressure to normal in patients with primary aldosteronism. Unfortunately, some 20 to 30 percent of patients with essential hypertension also become normotensive on spironolactone and it is impossible to distinguish this group without further laboratory testing. All patients with hypertension who respond to spironolactone with a significant fall in blood pressure, should have an evaluation for primary aldosteronism.

DIAGNOSTIC STUDIES IN HYPERTENSIVE PATIENTS WITH SPONTANEOUS OR EASILY INDUCIBLE HYPOKALEMIA

All saluretic agents, including thiazides and aldosterone antagonists are discontinued for 3 weeks, and the patients are then admitted to a hospital. They are given a diet containing 120 mEq of sodium and 50 mEq of potassium per day. Serum electrolytes are measured repeatedly throughout the period of hospitalization.

Excessive aldosterone production cannot be excluded without either measuring its secretion rate by isotope dilution or its urinary excretion as metabolites of aldosterone. On a 120 mEq sodium intake, 30–150 μg of aldosterone is normally secreted daily: 30 to 50 percent is excreted as urinary tetrahydroaldosterone-3-glucuronide, and 5 to 10 percent as the 18-monoglucuronide of unreduced aldosterone.

Aldosterone Secretion Rate (ASR)—Isotope Dilution Technique. A tracer dose (5 μCi) of ^{3}H-labeled aldosterone is injected intravenously. All urine passed in the succeeding 24 hours is collected, and the metabolites of aldosterone isolated. The specific activity (SA) of an isolated metabolite is determined and the secretion rate is then calculated:

$$\text{ASR} = \frac{\text{Injected dose of } ^{3}\text{H (cpm)}}{\text{SA of Urinary Metabolite}}$$

Aldosterone Excretion—Measurement of Urinary Metabolites. In the absence of liver or kidney disease, the production of aldosterone is increased if more than 16 μg of aldosterone monoglucuronide or more than 50 μg of tetrahydroaldosterone is excreted in 24 hours.

Unfortunately, a few patients who subsequently are found to have an aldosterone producing tumor at operation, secrete aldosterone at normal rates when examined. This is because spontaneous fluctuations in ASR can occur, allowing the rate to fall transiently into the normal range. The fact that in elderly subjects the normal range for ASR is lower than that for younger individuals, should also be taken into account when interpreting the results. The study should be repeated if there is any ambiguity.

Plasma Aldosterone Level; Deoxycorticosterone (DOCA) Suppression. The development of a radioimmunoassay to measure plasma aldosterone levels has been an important recent technical advance.[79] Aldosterone circulates in low concentrations in the plasma. Levels average 2 to 8 ng per 100 milliliters in recumbency and rise to 20 ng per 100 milliliters after 2 hours of the erect posture.

In primary aldosteronism plasma levels of aldosterone are increased in recumbency (12 ng per 100 milliliters) and do not fall after administration of DOCA (2 intramuscular injections of 10 mg each, 12 hours apart); in the absence of primary aldosteronism, the plasma aldosterone level decreases by a factor of 50 to 70 percent following DOCA.

Plasma Renin Activity (PRA). Blood samples for PRA are obtained in the morning when the patient is still recumbent, and then 4 hours later after the patient has been up and about. Measurement of PRA under basal conditions and then after the assumption of the upright posture (a maneuver which stimulates renin release) maximizes the detectable differences between normal subjects and patients with primary aldosteronism.

A subnormal PRA in recumbency which fails to increase significantly when the patient is up and active, is a highly reliable indication of the presence of primary aldosteronism. The PRA may be normally low in some patients with essential hypertension, but their aldosterone secretion rates are correspondingly low, and the PRA increases significantly in response to ambulation. Substantially elevated PRA after prolonged recumbency is a characteristic finding in hypertensive patients with secondary aldosteronism.

The simultaneous measurement of plasma renin activity and aldosterone concentration after at least 2 hours of erect posture provides valuable information as to the nature of a hypertensive disorder. After 2 hours of erect posture an increase of aldosterone concentration disproportionate to the stimulated plasma renin activity is diagnostic of primary aldosteronism (Fig. 2-5). In secondary aldosteronism, the increase in aldosterone concentration is proportionate to the plasma renin activity. Low renin hypertension exhibits both suppressed renin activity and appropriately reduced aldosterone levels as compared to normal subjects or patients with hypertension and normally responsive renin activity.

Spironolactone Response Test. Primary and secondary aldosteronism can also be distinguished by means of the Spironolactone Response Test.[65] There is quantitatively a much greater drop in blood pressure and in body weight in patients with primary aldosteronism treated with large doses of spironolactone for protracted periods, than in patients with secondary aldosteronism.

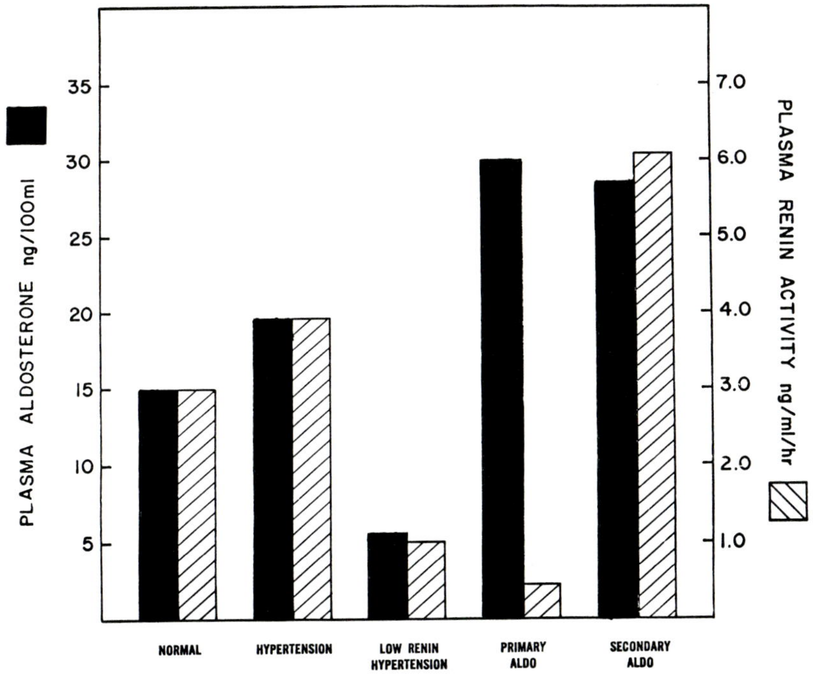

Fig. 2-5. Aldosterone concentration and renin activity in plasma after 2 hours of erect posture. (Courtesy of James C. Melby, M.D.)

The spironolactone response test is also useful in predicting the outcome of adrenal surgery for primary aldosteronism. A positive response to spironolactone is correlated with a good response to adrenalectomy.

The test is usually arranged to follow the in-hospital studies. Patients are dismissed on 400 mg of spironolactone per day for 3 to 5 weeks. Blood pressure, weight and electrolyte responses are followed closely during the period of treatment; the blood urea nitrogen (BUN) should also be checked periodically, since in patients with secondary aldosteronism a progressive rise of the BUN may be seen and the dose of spironolactone needs to be adjusted accordingly.

In 75 percent of patients with primary aldosteronism the diastolic blood pressure will drop more than 20 mm Hg. Weight loss at the end of the first week of therapy averages 2 to 3 kg. In patients with secondary aldosteronism there is no significant decrease in either blood pressure or weight.

Patients with an elevated ASR, with elevated plasma aldosterone levels not suppressible by DOCA, with a subnormal PRA and who exhibit a positive response to spironolactone therapy have a presumptive diagnosis of primary aldosteronism. These patients are readmitted to a hospital, the spironolactone is discontinued and tumor localization studies performed.

IDENTIFYING THE ADRENAL LESION IN PRIMARY ALDOSTERONISM

In recent years more and more patients with aldosterone excess and a low PRA have been found who do not conform to the classic pattern as described by Conn in 1955. These patients don't have typical, solitary aldosterone producing adenomas (APA), instead, their adrenals are hyperplastic—they have so-called "idiopathic" hyperaldosteronism (IHA). The reported incidence of IHA has varied widely, ranging from 18 percent to almost 50 percent of patients with primary aldosteronism. Of the 65 patients seen at Boston University Hospital between the years 1962 to 1972, 19 (30 percent) were found to have IHA.

All are agreed that the treatment of APA is removal by unilateral adrenalectomy, but there is less unanimity of opinion concerning the proper management of IHA. Bilateral total adrenalectomy has yielded satisfactory results. Other centers, however, have reported disillusionment with adrenalectomy citing that a high proportion of their patients treated in this way are not relieved of their hypertension, even though the aldosteronism and the potassium depletion may be corrected.[9] Some have suggested that if these patients could be accurately identified preoperatively, it might be preferable to advise no surgery and to treat them instead with antihypertensive medication.[9]

Recently, several groups in the United Kingdom have attempted to differentiate IHA from APA using a mathematical technique known as quadric analysis.[13] They have shown that by using a computer to simultaneously analyze multiple biochemical and clinical variables—including plasma aldosterone and electrolyte concentrations, PRA, blood pressure and age—they can, at least, retrospectively, separate tumor from nontumor groups. The reliability of the method to prospectively (preoperatively) distinguish between APA and IHA in individual patients with primary aldosteronism, has yet to be satisfactorily demonstrated.

Hyperplasia is probably best diagnosed by a process of exclusion; failure to identify or localize an adenoma preoperatively using the techniques discussed below, strongly suggest the presence of adrenal hyperplasia.

It should be emphasized that APA's are usually small, sometimes measuring just a few millimeters in diameter. As such they may not

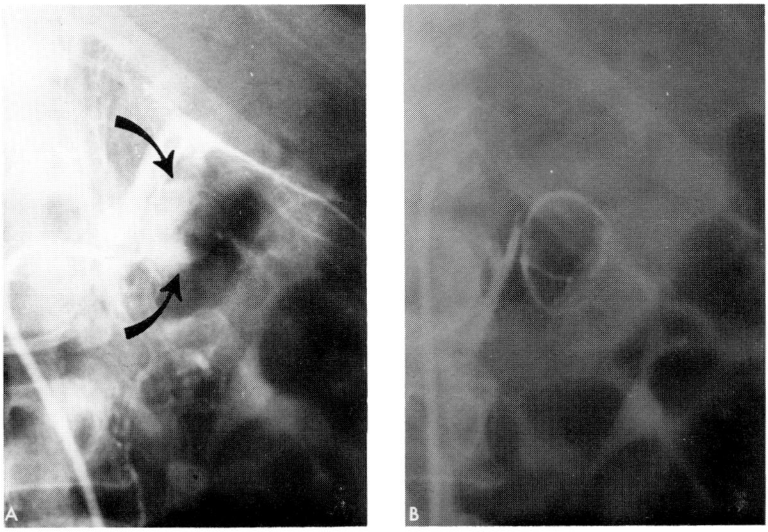

Fig. 2-6. A. Left middle adrenal arteriogram demonstrates a slightly vascular adenoma measuring 16 mm (arrows). B. Left adrenal venogram shows circumferential veins. (Reprinted by permission from Radiology 101:71, 1971.)

be palpable at the time of operation, and the surgeon who has not obtained preoperative localization studies may have to remove the normal gland in an effort to find the lesion. Even if it is not actually removed, the uninvolved gland may be devascularized in the process of freeing it up for palpation. In either event the end result is adrenal insufficiency and the necessity for life-long replacement therapy. This is an unnecessary medical risk and financial burden to the patient.

Adrenal Angiography and Aldosterone Assay of Adrenal Venous Blood. Adrenal arteriography by direct catheterization of adrenal arteries, when combined with selective vasoconstriction of the renal circulation, provides a reliable method for demonstrating the adrenal glands in spite of their variable blood supply. The adrenal arteries exhibit a striking unresponsiveness to epinephrine whereas the renal arteries show intense vasoconstriction. Consequently, post-epinephrine arteriograms of the renal and celiac arteries tend to visualize adrenal branches selectively. An experienced angiographer can demonstrate two-thirds or more of the adrenal gland in 80 percent of cases by adding the composite blushes from the various adrenal injections. An aldosteronoma usually appears as a sharply delineated avascular area within the densely opacified adrenal cortex (Fig. 2-6,A).

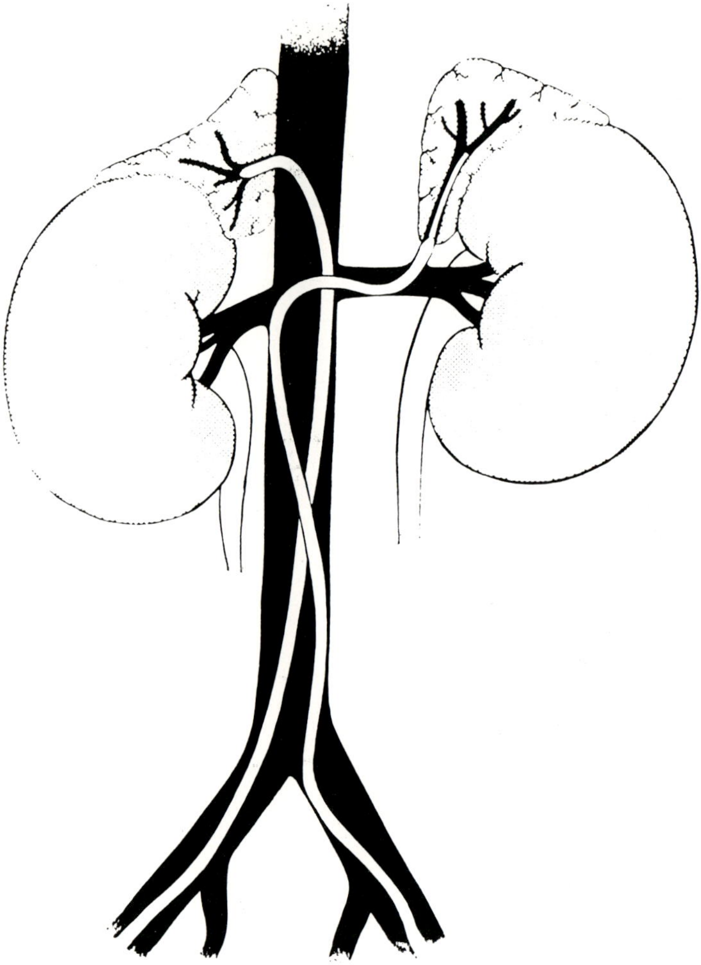

Fig. 2-7. Schematic illustration of bilateral adrenal-vein catheterization technique. (Reprinted by permission from NEJM 277:1050, 1967.)

Each adrenal gland is usually drained by a single vein. Selective catheterization of the right and left adrenal veins via a percutaneous, transfemoral approach permits not only angiographic studies but also collection of adrenal venous effluent for the purpose of comparing the plasma aldosterone concentrations from the two sides (Fig. 2-7). The venogram characteristically shows circumferential veins outlining the tumor and the absence of the normal reticular pattern associated with the right-angled branching of the adrenal veins (Fig. 2-6,B).

The procedure is not without risk, however. Intra-adrenal hemorrhage, which can lead to adrenal insufficiency, may result when contrast material is injected too forcefully. As Kahn[57] has pointed out, this complication is more likely to occur when trying to visualize a small tumor; the more difficult the visualization, the greater the volume of dye used, and the more forceful its injection.

Sampling of the venous effluent of both glands with measurement of aldosterone in the sampled blood enables lateralization of hyperfunction and localization of an APA.[68] If the aldosterone levels indicate hyperfunction on both sides a diagnosis of adrenocortical hyperplasia (IHA) is strongly suggested. We believe that an APA is identified if aldosterone levels in the effluent from the tumor-bearing gland are >2.0 μg percent, while the level is <0.5 μg percent in the venous effluent from the contralateral, noninvolved gland. IHA is present when the aldosterone levels in the venous effluent from both glands is >2.0 μg percent, or if on one side the effluent level is at least 1.0 μg percent while the other side is >2.0 μg percent.

The technique of adrenal vein catheterization with sampling requires considerable angiographic expertise. Even an experienced angiographer may fail to catheterize one or other adrenal vein (usually the right) in some 5 to 10 percent of cases. The value of the test is diminished under these circumstances, because its predictive accuracy is dependent on the comparison of aldosterone levels from both adrenal veins.

In practice, sampling of venous effluent is carried out before evaluation by angiography. Selective adrenal arteriography is performed as the next step and if good visualization of both glands is obtained one can dispense with the risky venogram. In a series of 38 cases of primary aldosteronism studied by adrenal angiography coupled with measurement of aldosterone in the venous effluent, a correct preoperative diagnosis of either tumor or hyperplasia was made consistently.

Photoscanning of Tumors after Administration of ^{131}I-19-Iodocholesterol. A technique which may eventually supplant adrenal angiography and adrenal venous sampling for tumor localization has recently been developed by Beierwaltes, Conn et al.[17] It is the technique of external photoscanning using ^{131}I-19-iodocholesterol. The labeled cholesterol is incorporated by the functioning adenoma to be used in the synthesis of aldosterone. Photoscans reveal a "hot spot" at the site of the adenoma (Fig. 2-8), whereas patients with bilateral hyperplasia exhibit a diffuse uptake by both adrenals. Interestingly, dexamethasone has been found to inhibit the uptake of labeled cholesterol in those cases with hyperplasia but it does not interfere with the uptake by the solitary ade-

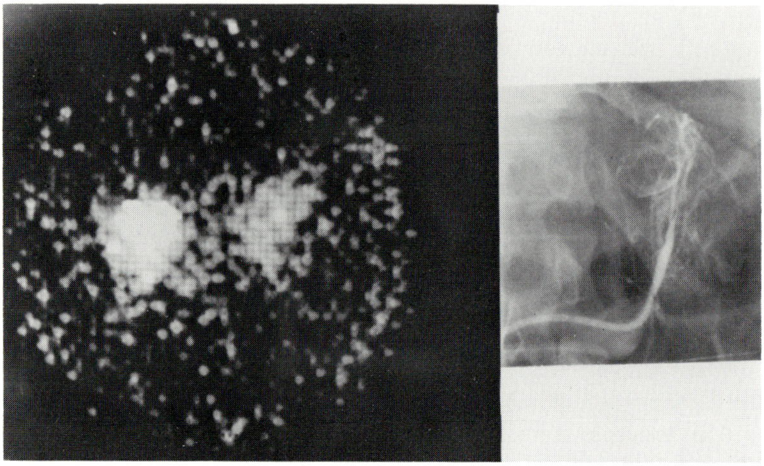

Fig. 2-8. Comparison of Anger camera scintiphoto (posterior view) with left adrenal venogram showing presence of a hyperfunctioning aldosterone secreting tumor of the left adrenal gland. (Reprinted by permission from Archives Int Med, 129:417, 1972; copyright 1972 Am Med Assn.)

noma. To date, the technique appears to have a satisfactory degree of resolution with few false positives. As a noninvasive approach to the problem of tumor localization it should prove of considerable value.

TREATMENT OF PRIMARY ALDOSTERONISM

The spectrum of pathologic findings in primary aldosteronism appears to have changed in recent years with proportionately more cases of adrenocortical hyperplasia (idiopathic hyperaldosteronism) being reported. In the Boston University Hospital experience, idiopathic hyperaldosteronism (IHA) now constitutes about one-third of the patients with the findings of primary aldosteronism; aldosterone-producing adenomas (APA) make up the remainder.

Removal of an APA results in cure of the hypertension and metabolic abnormalities in the majority of cases. The results of operative treatment in IHA have been much less encouraging. In our experience two-thirds of patients are still hypertensive following bilateral total adrenalectomy even though the metabolic consequences of aldosterone excess are corrected. Other investigators report even fewer cures for surgery in this condition and prefer instead to treat these patients nonoperatively with the aldosterone antagonist, spironolactone. It has even been suggested that spironolactone might be used to treat APA but the drug produces adverse reactions in a significant proportion of patients; including gastrointestinal disturbance, drowsiness, rashes, impotence, and gynecomastia; and there is always the remote possibility of a malignant neoplasm being present.[80]

Operative Treatment

INDICATIONS

All unilateral, solitary adrenocortical adenomas causing primary aldosteronism should be removed by unilateral adrenalectomy.

In the case of adrenocortical hyperplasia, bilateral total adrenalectomy results in a permanent cure of hypertension and metabolic abnormalities in about one-third of our patients, so that we continue to advocate primary surgical treatment in all cases where the patient is judged intelligent enough to conscientiously handle his own replacement therapy. Even though surgery may fail to restore the blood pressure to normal levels in the other two-thirds, most will exhibit some reduction in blood pressure and almost all will correct their metabolic abnormalities. In addition, even though the blood pressure may still be elevated, it will often be more amenable to treatment with conventional anti-hypertensive medication following bilateral adrenalectomy.[9]

PREOPERATIVE PREPARATION

Localization Studies. Localization studies are essential in all patients with primary aldosteronism. Most aldosteronomas are quite small, some measure a few millimeters in diameter. It is impossible to palpate these tiny lesions at surgery, even after extensive mobilization of the adrenal. If the surgeon knows beforehand the side on which the tumor is located, he can remove the offending gland even though he may not be able to see or feel the tumor. Even more important is the fact that the normal adrenal gland is not subjected to the risk of removal or devascularization in the course of a fruitless search for an adenoma.

The newer techniques of adrenal vein sampling, selective adrenal arteriography and iodocholesterol photoscanning can identify and lateralize aldosterone producing adenomas with a high degree of accuracy. The surgeon can therefore proceed with unilateral adrenalectomy from the posterior approach and remove the tumor without having to explore the uninvolved side.[28] If there is no lateralization of adrenal hyperfunction to either side and angiographic techniques fail to reveal a discrete lesion, adrenocortical hyperplasia is most probably present and bilateral total adrenalectomy will be necessary if the patient does not respond to spironolactone treatment. Some recommend surgery for all patients with hyperplasia.

Spironolactone Pretreatment. Surgery in the presence of hypokalemia is known to carry a greater risk. Spironolactone, in a daily dose of 300–400 mg for 1 to 2 weeks prior to surgery, taken together with oral potassium supplements (about 50 mEq per day), substantially corrects both the hypertension and the potassium deficiency of primary aldosteronism and significantly reduces the incidence of operative and postoperative complications, such as cardiac irregularities and paralytic ileus.[71] Pretreatment with spironolactone may also attenuate the period of postoperative aldosterone deficiency which otherwise results from prolonged suppression of the renin–angiotensin system.

OPERATIVE APPROACH

For years, one of the most controversial aspects in the treatment of primary aldosteronism was whether or not to operate from the posterior or anterior approach.[27] Now that preoperative localization studies have been established as a routine, and it is no longer necessary to explore both adrenals in all cases, the argument has been largely resolved in favor of the posterior approach.

Unilateral adrenalectomy can be performed with less morbidity and mortality from the posterior approach, postoperative pain is less troublesome, pulmonary complications are infrequent and paralytic ileus is rarely a problem. With removal of the 12th rib, the exposure of the adrenal is excellent and there is no need for extensive mobilization and retraction of the surrounding viscera. Using the posterior approach, bilateral total adrenalectomy, when indicated, can be accomplished efficiently by two operating teams working simultaneously on opposite sides of the table.

Surgery should not be undertaken without the benefit of preoperative localization studies, but if all attempts at localization have failed, many advocate that the left adrenal be explored first (there is a statistically higher chance of finding an adenoma on the left). If an adenoma is found, the gland is removed; if the gland is enlarged or nodular, it should also be removed along with the gland on the right hand side; if the left adrenal, however, is normal by inspection and palpation, the gland on the right should then be explored carefully. If the right adrenal is found to contain an adenoma, it is removed but in the event that it also appears to be normal, we would perform bilateral total adrenalectomy (*provided* the diagnosis of primary aldosteronism has been firmly established preoperatively).

Postoperative Care

If bilateral adrenalectomy is to be performed for IHA, the patient is given 50 mg of cortisol intramuscularly on call to the operating room. An intravenous infusion of cortisol, at 15 mg per hour, is begun with the dissection of the adrenals. Postoperatively the infusion is continued at 10 mg per hour; intramuscular supplementation with an additional 50 mg every 8 hours is ordered to guard against the possibility of undetected infiltration of the intravenous line. The subsequent dosage schedule is outlined in the section Posterior Approach to Adrenalectomy; in patients operated on for primary aldosteronism the maintenance dose of cortisol is about 20 to 30 mg per day. These dosages are predicated upon the experimentally supported estimate that the normal adrenals produce approximately 10 to 20 mg of cortisol per day. A small dose 0.05–0.1 mg) of fluorohydrocortisone, a synthetic mineralocorticoid, will be required to regulate sodium metabolism.

Following unilateral adrenalectomy for APA, no special measures are required if the patient has been adequately prepared preoperatively with spironolactone. When spironolactone has not been given, there is a definite risk of adrenal insufficiency following surgery, particularly if a good sodium intake is not maintained. Salt retention in these patients is poor due to the fact that the remaining adrenal gland is suppressed in its ability to secrete aldosterone for some time after removal of the functioning tumor.

Results of Operative Treatment

The blood pressure usually reverts to normal within a matter of weeks following removal of an APA. Unfortunately, a few patients experience a prolonged normotensive interval after the operation only to become hypertensive again within 5 years. The reasons are obscure, but a partial explanation may be found in the fact that a significant proportion of patients with primary aldosteronism report a strong family history of essential hypertension.[67] Some patients may have irreversible nephrosclerosis at the time of diagnosis, but considering the usual benign course of hypertension in primary aldosteronism, this situation must be uncommon.

At Boston University Hospital 13 of 19 patients (68 percent) with bilateral diffuse hyperplasia of the adrenal glands were hypertensive again one year after bilateral total adrenalectomy, even though their sodium and potassium metabolism remained normal in all cases. Followed over a 5-year period, however, there has been no increasing incidence of recurrent hypertension in this group. Thus it seems that a surgical cure in cases of IHA, if obtained, will be permanent.

Nonoperative Treatment

Spironolactone is a steroidal lactone which competes at the renal tubular cell to inhibit aldosterone and block sodium reabsorption. It has been used successfully in the long term treatment of primary aldosteronism when the underlying cause is IHA. It may also be used in patients with APA who have a definite contraindication to surgery, such as a recent myocardial infarction or severe, irreversible pulmonary disease.

The drug may be given either alone, when it is used in high doses (200-400 mg per day), or in combination with other antihypertensive agents when it can be used in a smaller dose; it potentiates the action of most of the currently used antihypertensive agents. With the larger dose, side effects are common and in the case of male patients, gynecomastia and impotence may seriously limit its use. Spironolactone may cause menstrual irregularities in females but nevertheless is usually regarded as an acceptable mode of prolonged therapy.

If the patient is judged intelligent enough to conscientiously handle his own steroid replacement therapy, then bilateral adrenalectomy is the preferred treatment for IHA in our opinion. Patients with limited intelligence, alcoholism or psychiatric disability cannot be managed with bilateral total adrenalectomy under any circumstances, for obvious reasons.

CUSHING'S SYNDROME

Diagnosis

Cushing's syndrome is an uncommon but potentially lethal metabolic derangement caused by the overproduction of cortisol.

Approximately 70 percent of all cases are due to bilateral adrenocortical hyperplasia resulting from an increased secretion of adrenocorticotrophin (ACTH) by the pituitary (classical Cushing's disease).

ACTH is also secreted by a number of benign and malignant tumors of nonendocrine origin resulting in adrenocortical hyperplasia.

The so-called 'ectopic ACTH syndrome' accounts for approximately 5 percent of all cases of Cushing's syndrome.

About 25 percent of patients with Cushing's syndrome have adrenal tumors; in adults, the majority are benign adenomas, whereas in children carcinomas predominate. The latter are usually highly malignant and rapidly fatal.

CLINICAL FEATURES OF CUSHING'S SYNDROME

When clinical manifestations are florid and the condition advanced, the diagnosis of Cushing's syndrome presents little difficulty. In approximately half of the 30 cases studied by Scott[78] and his colleagues, the diagnosis of Cushing's syndrome was obvious before special endocrine studies were performed, while in the other half the special tests clearly established the diagnosis. The major features of the syndrome reflect the exaggerated activities of cortisol; they are listed in the accompanying table (Table 1-1).

Diagnostic problems are presented by (1) early or mild forms of the disease, when signs may be minimal and symptoms non-specific; (2) patients with ectopic ACTH syndrome, in whom the clinical picture of Cushing's syndrome is overshadowed by the manifestations of disseminated malignancy; and (3) obese, hirsute women, who may be impossible to distinguish from Cushing's syndrome on clinical grounds.

Cushing's disease, i.e., that due to hypersecretion of pituitary ACTH, accounts for the vast majority of cases. It is seen predominantly in young adults with a peak incidence in the third and fourth decades of life. Women are affected more often than men, the ratio being about 4:1. Some of these patients have adenomas of the anterior pituitary; the exact incidence is unknown, but pituitary tumors large enough to be visualized radiologically have been reported in as many as 20 percent. Sometimes these tumors will enlarge enough to cause field defects; on rare occasions they are locally invasive. Whether or not there is an obvious pituitary tumor, the basic defect in Cushing's syndrome is believed to lie at the hypothalamic or cerebral level.

Cushing's syndrome due to the ectopic secretion of ACTH has been shown to occur with a wide variety of benign and malignant neoplasms of the lung, thymus, breast, prostate, ovary, and gastrointestinal tract. Most often a highly malignant lesion is responsible, and the most common of these is a bronchial carcinoma of the oat cell type. Patients with ectopic ACTH syndrome usually have generalized tissue wasting and weight loss with widespread, disseminated metastases; sometimes the only manifestation of their Cushing's syndrome is hypokalemic alkalosis.

Table 1–1
Clinical Manifestations in Cushing's Syndrome

Truncal obesity	95%
Hypertension	85%
Glucosuria and decreased glucose tolerance	80%
Menstrual and sexual dysfunction	75%
Hirsutism and acne	70%
Striae	70%
Muscle weakness	65%
Osteoporosis	55%
Easy bruisability	55%
Poor wound healing	55%
Psychiatric disturbances	50%
Edema, hypokalemic alkalosis	40%
Polyuria	15%

These tumors may secrete other peptide hormones in addition to ACTH; hyperpigmentation due to ectopic secretion of MSH (melanocyte-stimulating hormone) is one of the most common accompaniments.[8]

Cushing's syndrome due to adrenal carcinoma is often associated with pronounced virilization because of increased 17-ketosteroid excretion.[55] The combination of hirsutes, acne and amenorrhea with rapidly progressive Cushing's syndrome in a younger, female patient with elevated 17-ketosteroid excretion is very suggestive of adrenal carcinoma. Some carcinomas are such inefficient synthesizers of steroid, that before the patient has clinically recognizable Cushing's syndrome, the tumor has enlarged sufficiently to be palpable through the body wall.

SCREENING TESTS FOR CUSHING'S SYNDROME

Plasma Cortisol and Circadian Rhythm Studies. Normally, the secretion of ACTH and cortisol varies throughout the day (circadian rhythm), following a predictable diurnal rhythm with plasma levels maximal at about the time of waking and minimal at about the time of going to sleep (Fig. 2-9). In Cushing's syndrome the circadian rhythm is lost. This can be demonstrated by measurement of plasma cortisol at 8 a.m. and again at 8 p.m. In normal subjects blood cortisol levels vary between 5 and 30 μg per 100 milliliters at 8 a.m. and fall to below 10 μg per 100 milliliters by 8 p.m. Patients with early Cushing's syndrome may have normal or high-normal plasma cortisol levels at

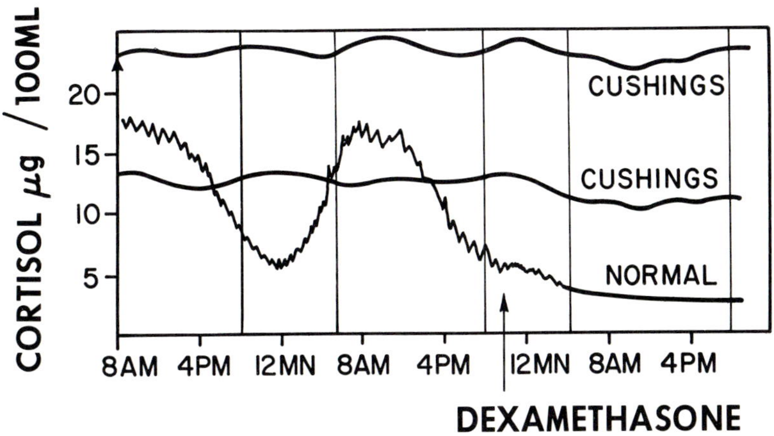

Fig. 2-9. A diurnal rhythm in cortisol secretion is present in a normal subject but is lacking in 2 patients with Cushing's syndrome. A small dose of dexamethasone given at midnight suppresses the a.m. plasma cortisol level in the normal subject but not in those with Cushing's syndrome.

8 a.m., but they show no reduction of this level in the evening. Melby[66] has emphasized the importance of this phenomenon in explaining the appearance of Cushing's syndrome when basal cortisol production rate is only moderately increased. Demonstration of the absence of a diurnal rhythm in plasma cortisol levels is the single most important test in the diagnosis of Cushing's syndrome.

Urinary Excretion of 17-hydroxycorticosteroids and Free Cortisol. Cortisol is metabolized by the liver. About 50 percent of metabolites are excreted in the urine as 17-hydroxycorticosteroids (17-OHCS), where they can be measured by a specific chromogen reaction. Males excrete from 2 to 10 mg per 24 hours, females slightly less. For years, determination of the 24-hour urinary excretion of 17-OHCS was a mainstay in the laboratory diagnosis of Cushing's syndrome. Actually, however, the correlation between urinary 17-OHCS excretion and the production of cortisol is not consistent; the cortisol secretion rate (CSR) may be elevated in the presence of normal urinary 17-OHCS.

Urinary free cortisol excretion gives a better correlation with CSR and is usually elevated in all forms of Cushing's syndrome. The normal value for urinary free cortisol excretion is between 80 to 400 μg per day.

Cortisol Secretion Rate (CSR). The CSR is an accurate index of adrenal secretory activity. It can be measured directly by isotope dilution methods. A tracer dose of ^{3}H-labeled cortisol is injected intravenously and all urine passed in the succeeding 24 hours is collected. The metabolites of cortisol are isolated by thin-layer chromatography and the specific activity (SA) of a reduced glucuronic acid conjugate of cortisol is determined. The secretion rate is then calculated:

$$\text{CSR} = \frac{\text{Injected dose of } ^3\text{H (cpm)}}{\text{SA of Urinary Metabolite}}.$$

The basal secretion of cortisol varies from 10 to 28 mg per 24 hours. Adrenal secretory activity can fluctuate widely in patients with Cushing's syndrome, so that some patients may have a normal secretion rate when studied. The determination should be repeated if there is any ambiguity.

Low Dose Dexamethasone Suppression Test. Small doses of exogenous cortisol or synthetic cortisol derivatives (dexamethasone) suppress the pituitary-adrenal axis to inhibit cortisol secretion in the normal subject but not in the patient with Cushing's syndrome (Fig. 2-9). One mg of dexamethasone taken at midnight will normally suppress the 8 a.m. blood cortisol concentration to a value of 5 μg per 100 milliliters or below, whereas patients with Cushing's syndrome show either no suppression whatsoever, or, more commonly, partial but incomplete suppression.

This test is a useful screening test for Cushing's syndrome which has proved consistently reliable in outpatient populations. Some false positives have been reported when the test is applied in hospitalized patients, however, presumably because the level of anxiety and stress in these patients is sometimes sufficient to obliterate the suppressive effect of a single, small dose of dexamethasone. In this situation the test is best repeated using a dose of 0.5 mg of dexamethasone which is given every 6 hours for 48 hours. Plasma cortisol is sampled each morning, before, during and after the test.

TESTS TO ESTABLISH THE ETIOLOGY OF CUSHING'S SYNDROME

Once the diagnosis of Cushing's syndrome has been established by demonstration of increased cortisol production, special laboratory tests can be carried out to determine the etiology.

High Dose Dexamethasone Suppression Test. Dexamethasone in a dose of 2 mg every 6 hours for 2 days will suppress plasma cortisol in patients with adrenal hyperplasia due to excess pituitary ACTH, but will usually fail to suppress cortisol levels in patients with adrenal tumors or ectopic ACTH production.

Metyrapone Test. Metyrapone inhibits 11-β hydroxylation (see Fig. 2-15) to block the final step in the synthesis of cortisol; the immediate precursor, 11-deoxycortisol (compound S), is secreted instead. In normal subjects ACTH is secreted by the hypothalamic–pituitary axis when the plasma cortisol falls below a critical level and this in turn leads to increased production of compound S by the adrenal cortex. Increased S production is reflected in an increased urinary 17-OHCS excretion and also in an increased level of plasma S measured by radioimmunoassay.

A single, large dose of metyrapone ($\sim$30 mg/kg) is given at midnight and plasma S determined at 8 a.m. the following morning.[81] In normal subjects the plasma S will be increased from a normal level or less than 1 μg per 100 milliliters to a level of 7 to 18 μg per 100 milliliters. In patients with Cushing's disease there is an exaggerated plasma S and urinary 17-OHCS response to metyrapone. By contrast, patients with adrenal tumors and most patients with the ectopic ACTH syndrome will have chronically suppressed pituitary function and therefore fail to release ACTH in response to metyrapone; the plasma S remains unchanged.

ACTH Stimulation Test. The adrenal hyperplasia of Cushing's disease will respond to exogenous ACTH by an increase in plasma cortisol and urinary 17-OHCS. Twenty-five USP units of ACTH are given by rapid intravenous injection and blood samples are collected for cortisol analysis, before injection of ACTH and two hours afterwards.

In the ectopic ACTH syndrome the adrenals are usually maximally stimulated and fail to respond. Most adrenal tumors also show no response; unfortunately, some do; approximately 50 percent of adenomas and also some carcinomas. The unpredictability of the response to ACTH by adrenal tumors makes this a poor test for differentiating the various etiologic subtypes of Cushing's syndrome.

Plasma ACTH Assay. A reliable radioimmunoassay for ACTH has been developed only recently. It is not yet generally available, but in time it should prove to be an extremely useful tool in differential diagnosis.

Patients whose adrenal hyperfunction does not suppress with high doses of dexamethasone (i.e., adrenal tumors and ectopic ACTH syndrome) can be distinguished by plasma ACTH assay: Adrenal tumors

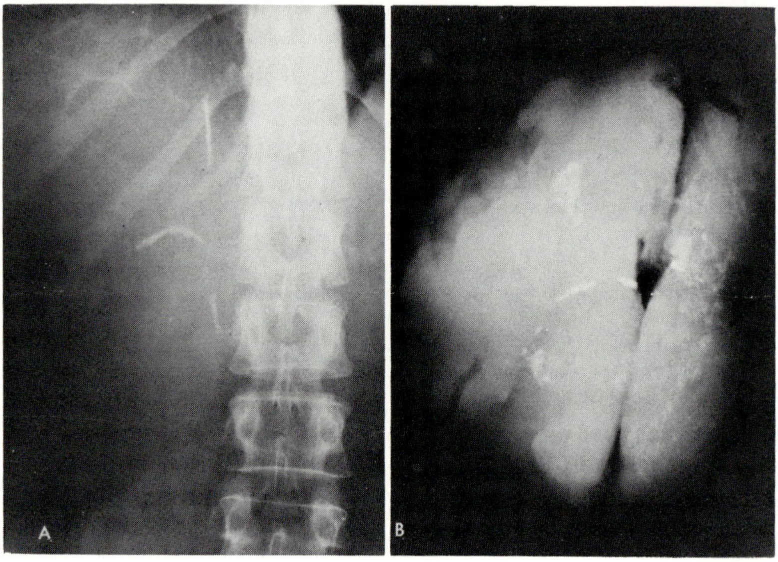

Fig. 2-10. A. Dense bands of calcification in a large right adrenal cortical carcinoma. The calcium is usually deposited in the more necrotic portions of the tumor, and fails to reflect its full size. B. Radiograph of resected specimen. (Reprinted by permission from Radiol Clin N Am 5:221, 1967.)

suppress ACTH secretion by the pituitary so that plasma levels of ACTH are usually unmeasurable, whereas the ectopic ACTH syndrome is associated with high levels of ACTH.

Urinary 17-Ketosteroids (17-KS). The finding of hypersecretion of adrenal adrogens with increased 17-ketosteroid excretion in the urine is of value in the recognition of adrenal cortical carcinoma.[55] Normal 24-hour urinary 17-KS excretion averages 10 $\pm$ 5 mg for adult females and 15 $\pm$ 5 mg for males. While moderate increases in 17-KS excretion may occur in many patients with Cushing's syndrome due to hyperplasia, adenoma or the ectopic production of ACTH, striking increases (in the range of 40 to 100 mg per 24 hours) are characteristic only of adrenal carcinoma.

Identifying the Adrenal Lesion in Cushing's Syndrome. X-ray studies of the skull with views of the sella turcica should be performed as a routine in patients with Cushing's syndrome. Enlargement or erosion of the sella suggests a pituitary tumor with accompanying adrenal hyperplasia.

An intravenous pyelogram may show unilateral renal displacement

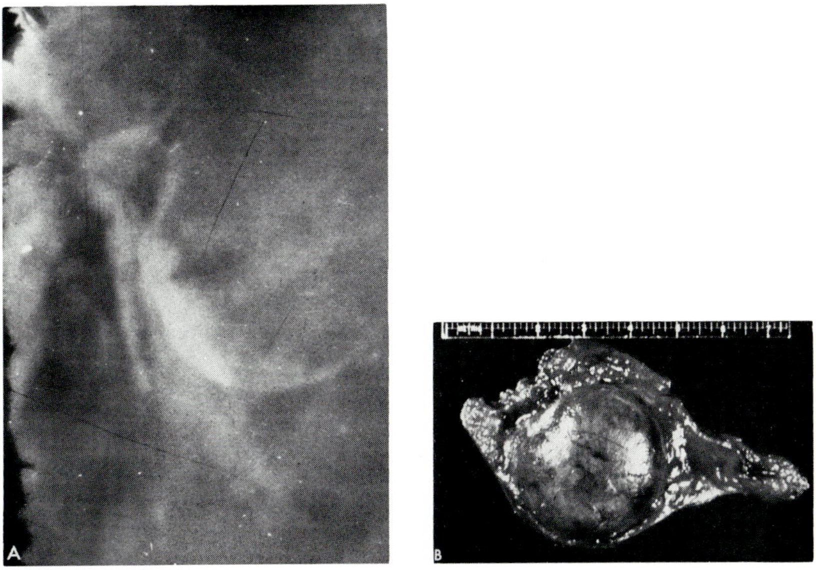

Fig. 2-11. A. Adrenal cortical adenoma causing Cushing's syndrome demonstrated by middle adrenal arteriography of the left side. B. Gross specimen of lesion in A. (Reprinted by permission from Am J Surg 117:480, 1969.)

in cases of adrenal tumor and when combined with nephrotomography the tumor itself can often be outlined. The presence of calcium in the mass is highly suggestive of carcinoma[56] (Fig. 2-10).

When the intravenous pyelogram fails to reveal a tumor, selective adrenal arteriography is the most useful tool in making the diagnosis. Even when the diagnosis of adrenal tumor seems fairly certain, an arte-

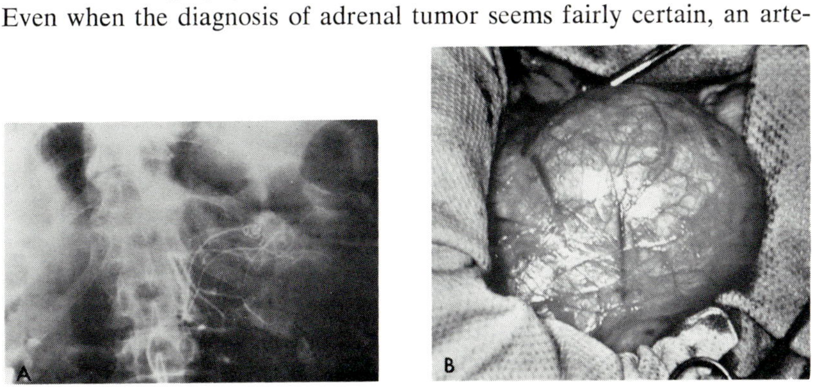

Fig. 2-12. A. Malignant adrenal tumor demonstrated by left middle adrenal arteriogram. B. Operative photograph of lesion in A. (Reprinted by permission from Am J Surg 117:480, 1969.)

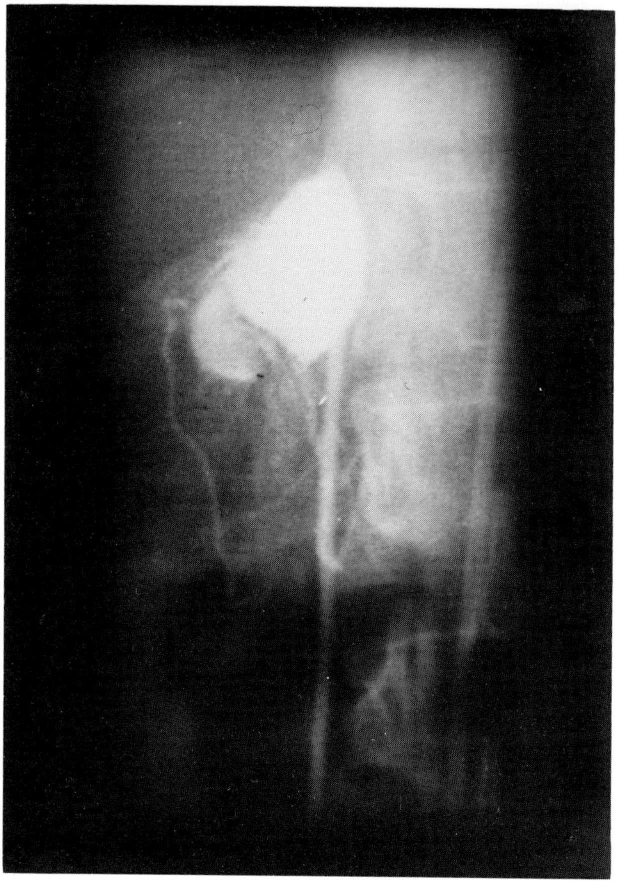

Fig. 2-13. Venogram demonstrating extravasation of contrast medium into the right adrenal gland.

riogram will provide a useful "road map" for the surgeon by outlining the blood supply to the tumor (Figs. 2-11 and 2-12).

Some surgeons feel adrenal venography is unwise in patients with Cushing's syndrome. The risk of dye extravasation and adrenal hemorrhage secondary to adrenal vein catheterization in these patients is high; perhaps because of the undue fragility of the adrenal capillaries (Fig. 2-13). Increased capillary fragility in Cushing's syndrome is a generalized phenomenon, as is evidenced by the frequent appearance of skin bruises after minimal or unnoticed trauma.

Radioiodinated cholesterol is taken up by the adrenal glands and utilized in the synthesis of corticosteroids. Rectilinear scanning or

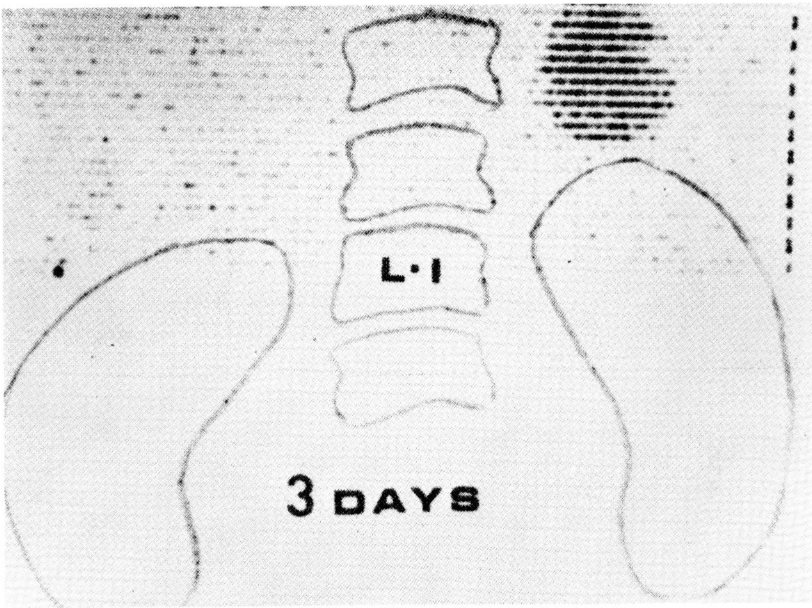

Fig. 2-14. Scintillation scan of the adrenal areas three days after administration of ^{131}I-19-iodocholesterol to a patient with Cushing's syndrome due to a right adrenal adenoma. The view is from the posterior aspect and uptake of the isotope by the adenoma is seen. (Reprinted by permission from the NEJM 285:1387, 1971.)

gamma-camera imaging of the adrenals after injection of ^{131}I-19-iodocholesterol permits localization of adrenal tumors and their differentiation from bilateral adrenocortical hyperplasia.[62] A functioning tumor shows up as a "hot spot" on one side (Fig. 2-14); hyperplasia is characterized by an increased concentration of radioactivity bilaterally. Although there has been only limited experience with the new method, resolution appears to be excellent, and, as a noninvasive technique, it would seem to have obvious advantages over adrenal angiography.

Treatment of Cushing's Syndrome

GENERAL CONSIDERATIONS

The treatment of Cushing's syndrome depends critically upon the etiology. Most commonly the syndrome results from adrenal cortical hyperplasia, but it may also result from a benign adrenal cortical tumor or from adrenal cortical carcinoma. As indicated elsewhere, the appropriate use of physiologic testing can lead to a correct preoperative diagnosis with great consistency. There is uniform agreement that the treatment of choice with benign adrenal cortical tumor and Cushings's syndrome is unilateral adrenalectomy. If the tumor has been localized preoperatively it can be approached conveniently by the posterior approach, although the anterior approach is preferred by some. Adrenalectomy is also the treatment of choice in adrenal cortical carcinoma. However, it is desirable in this case to include a large segment of the periadrenal fat. Metastasis to the opposite adrenal is a common occurrence, so that bilateral adrenalectomy is often indicated. In addition, on the right side there is frequently invasion of the vena cava by the tumor, which may necessitate resection of a portion of vena cava and insertion of a venous patch graft. Because of these considerations, the anterior approach to the adrenals is preferable in cases of carcinoma. Since palliation with drugs such as *O,p′*DDD may be limited by the tolerance of patients and since the dose required depends on the amount of functional tissue present, it appears desirable to resect all tumor possible even if cure seems unattainable.

There is much less general agreement concerning the treatment of adrenal hyperplasia with Cushing's syndrome. In those few cases in which a pituitary tumor can be demonstrated, a transsphenoidal approach to the pituitary with resection of the tumor is indicated. If there is ectopic production of ACTH by an oatcell carcinoma, radiotherapy of the tumor appears to be the treatment of choice. In most cases however, increased release of ACTH by the pituitary stems from aberrant central neural control. If the syndrome is not severe, it is common practice to attempt to reduce pituitary function by external radiation of the pituitary. The dose normally used varies between 4000 and 5000 rads.[75] This treatment leads to normal secretion of cortisol only about one-fourth of the time, but may improve the syndrome in other cases. Panhypopituitarism is rare with this degree of radiation. The success rate has been improved recently by use of radiation with a proton beam to deliver 9000 to 10,000 rads. However, in this case hypopituitarism, seizures and oculomotor palsies may occur.[25] Surgical hypophysectomy is generally considered undesirable in Cushing's disease without pituitary tumor since it may not cure the disease if it is incomplete, and since panhypopituitarism is an invariable result if it is complete. Since most of the patients are females of childbearing age, hypopituitarism is generally considered an unwarranted sequel. In addition, diabetes insipidus occurs not uncommonly and presents special problems of control.

Because of these considerations it is generally agreed that surgery on the hyperplastic adrenals is appropriate. Recently there have been attempts to control the syndrome medically by the use of inhibitors of synthesis of cortisol such as *O,p′*DDD or aminoglutethamide. These agents have been used only experimentally in the treatment of Cushing's syndrome with hyperplasia and are not generally accepted. They are useful adjuncts, however, in the treatment of inoperable carcinoma of the adrenal cortex.

The only generally satisfactory treatment of adrenal corticol hyperplasia in most cases is bilateral total adrenalectomy. Previous attempts to leave an adrenal remnant have led almost uniformly to recurrent adrenal hyperplasia in the remnant. In patients with severe Cushing's syndrome the tissue weakness and waste resulting from the catabolic action of cortisol may present a nutritional problem. In some cases patients have been treated for six months or more with *O,p′*DDD to inhibit synthesis of cortisol and to allow tissue regeneration. Furthermore, in some cases which present with severe hypokalemia, the use of spironolactone as an adjunct to therapy is also indicated to allow preoperative repletion of potassium. Bilateral adrenalectomy can be accomplished either by the posterior approach using two teams to reduce operative time or by the anterior approach. The choice is a matter of individual preference and the authors of this volume disagree among themselves. Whichever approach is used, meticulous control of the adrenal veins and protection of the inferior vena cava are critical, since the most common cause of death is postoperative hemorrhage. In addition, the massively overweight patient with Cushing's syndrome presents a problem in postoperative mobilization. Early ambulation is essential to prevent both thromboembolic phenomena and pulmonary complications.

Although most patients with Cushing's syndrome do not present with a pituitary tumor, approximately one patient in 10 will develop a chromophobe adenoma of the pituitary following adrenalectomy. The adenoma appears to possess low-grade malignancy and is first suspected by the develoment of progressive hyperpigmentation (Nelson's Syndrome).[73] Such tumors have been found to contain not only large quantities of ACTH, but also large quantities of MSH as well. The treatment of Nelson's Syndrome is surgical resection of the pituitary.

STEROID THERAPY IN CUSHING'S SYNDROME

All patients with Cushing's syndrome require intraoperative steroid therapy, even when only a single adrenal is being resected for tumor. This is the case because excess secretion of cortisol by the tumor has led to suppression of release of ACTH by the pituitary and thus to involution of the opposite adrenal. In this case, some months are commonly required before the remaining adrenal will develop normal function. There are several options for preoperative and intraoperative steroid therapy. Some surgeons prefer to begin steroid therapy with the surgery by giving 100 mg of cortisol intravenously during the operation, preferably by bolus injection. Three hundred milligrams of cortisol represents the average requirement during the operative day. Alternatively, the patient can be prepared with oral or intramuscular steroids. These should be given at the rate of 100 mg of cortisol or its equivalent the night before surgery and the morning of surgery. Two mg of dexamethasone appears convenient to us since it is available in both oral form for the night dose and intramuscular form for the morning dose. Dexamethasone achieves its peak action at 6 hours so that this schedule allows a complete and adequate coverage of the intraoperative period. The use of this regimen obviates the need for intravenous infusion of steroid during surgery as well as the possibility that adrenal cortical insufficiency will occur at this time. Steroid therapy is reduced postoperatively by 50 percent per day until one arrives at a maintenance dose of steroid. The patient with Cushing's syndrome commonly requires greater than the minimum dose of steroid for some weeks. In our experience the average patient requires 50 to 100 mg of cortisone per day during this time. If bilateral adrenalectomy is carried out the patient will also require 0.1 mg per day of 9α-fluorocortisol to compensate for the absence of aldosterone. This is available only in the oral form, however if hypotension is to be avoided, it is essential therefore on the day of surgery to compensate by intravenous therapy for the inevitable loss of sodium. Ultimately the patient will be brought into equilibrium with the standard maintenance dose of steroid, which is 37.5 mg per day of cortisone and 0.1 mg per day of 9α-fluorocortisol.

It is essential that the patient with adrenal insufficiency be educated to a reasonable extent in the nature of this problem. The patient should be instructed to double the dose of cortisone or its equivalent in the presence of even a mild illness, and to seek medical attention in the presence of severe illness. The patient should also carry some sort of medical identification indicating that in the event of injury or sudden illness he or she should be given 100 mg of soluble cortisol immediately intravenously.

ADRENOGENITAL SYNDROMES, CARCINOMA OF THE ADRENAL CORTEX

Diagnosis

Adrenogenital syndromes are characterized by virilization which is produced by an excessive secretion of adrenal androgens.

The adrenal cortex normally secretes a number of androgenic substances, including the weakly androgenic 17-ketosteroids (17-KS); dehydroepiandrosterone (DHA), etiocholanolone, androsterone, and their 11-oxy derivatives, and small amounts of the more potent androgen, testosterone. An excess of androgen is produced by adrenocortical tumors (usually carcinomas), or by bilateral adrenocortical hyperplasia.

BILATERAL ADRENOCORTICAL HYPERPLASIA

The adrenogenital syndrome in infants and young children is secondary to bilateral adrenocortical hyperplasia in almost all cases. These children are born with an inherited deficiency of one of the five enzymes involved in the biosynthesis of cortisol (Fig. 2-15).

In over 95 percent of cases hydroxylation at the C-21 position of the steroid nucleus is deficient and 17-hydroxyprogesterone cannot be converted into cortisol; it is diverted instead into metabolic pathways leading to the formation of 17 ketosteroids (Fig. 2-16). The shortage of cortisol evokes an increased secretion of adrenocorticotrophin (ACTH) which, in turn, produces adrenocortical hyperplasia. There is increased formation and accumulation of 17-hydroxyprogesterone and its androgenic metabolites. Fortunately, the deficiency of 21-hydroxylase is only partial in most cases so that the adrenals are able to produce enough aldosterone to minimize sodium loss and enough cortisol to avert adrenal insufficiency. When the enzyme defect is complete, the condition must be recognized within the first few days of life, before a salt-losing crisis supervenes.

A deficiency of the enzyme, 11-hydroxylase, will cause not only overproduction of adrenal androgen but also excess deoxycorticosterone, a salt-retaining steroid. Hypertension and genital abnormalities co-exist in these children.

Deficiencies of the remaining 3 enzymes (20,22 desmolase, 3 hydroxysteroid dehydrogenase and 17 hydroxylase) are extremely rare. Infants afflicted with these conditions do not survive their extreme, total adrenocortical insufficiency.

Clinical Features of 21-Hydroxylase Deficiency. Most females with adrenogenital syndrome due to enzyme defect will be identified at birth or soon after. Their external genitalia, under the influence of excess adrenal androgens, have been induced to differentiate in a masculinized fashion with enlargement of the clitoris and variable fusion of the labioscrotal folds. It should be noted however, that internal genital ductal differentiation occurs before the adrenal gland is functionally developed, so that the uterus, tubes, and ovaries are normal. Where necessary, appropriate restorative surgery to the external genitalia makes

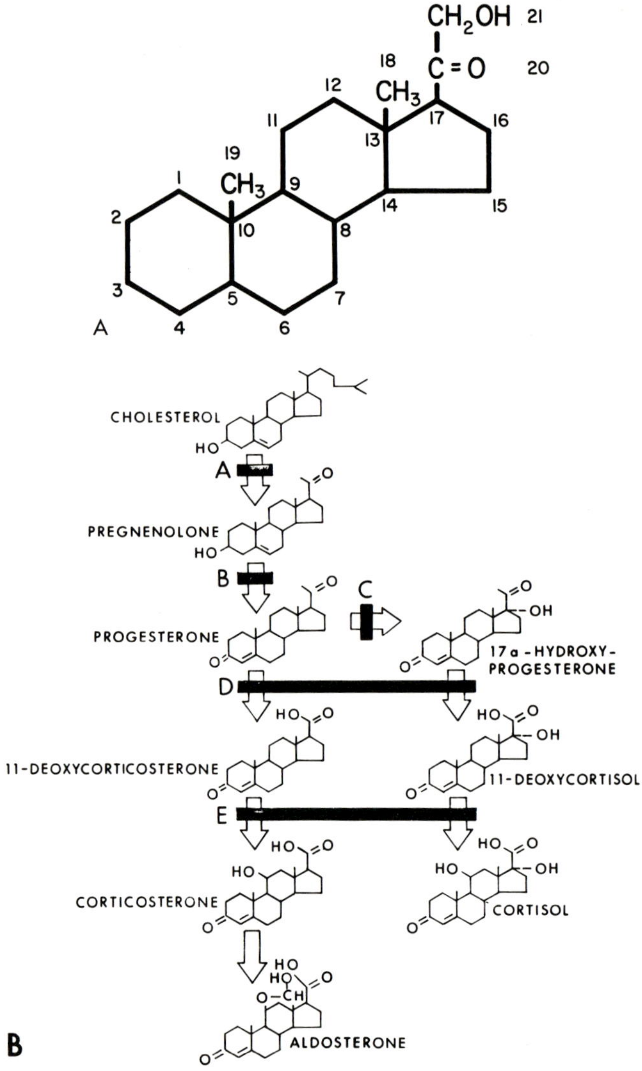

Fig. 2-15. A. Conventional numbering of carbon atom positions on the steroid molecule is shown. B. Biosynthetic pathway of adrenal steroids. Enzymatic "block" deficits can occur at A (desmolase), B (dehydrogenase), C (17-hydroxylase), D (21-hydroxylase), and E (11-hydroxylase).

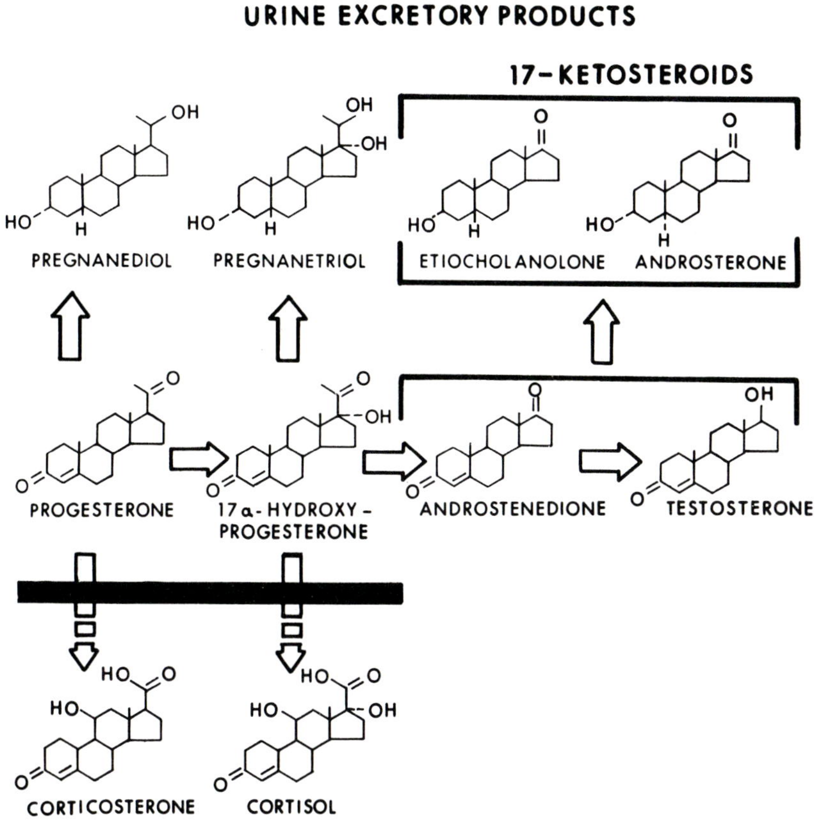

Fig. 2-16. Congenital adrenal hyperplasia due to 21-hydroxylase deficiency. Block produces deficits in corticosterone and cortisol, and increases urine excretory metabolites of progesterone, 17-hydroxyprogesterone, androstenedione, and testosterone.

it possible for these patients to realize complete femininity, including child bearing.

Sometimes the defect in C-21 hydroxylation is so mild that the affected individuals reach adult life without recognition or treatment of their condition. These women are characteristically obese but their habitus is feminine; usually their only abnormality is increased hirsutism, although sometimes they will have amenorrhea.

Occasionally, the degree of masculinization of the external genitalia is so great as to suggest the male gender, and the child is mistakenly reared as a boy. Without treatment, the female infant grows rapidly, acquires sexual hair and goes on to develop acne, deepening of the voice, further enlargement of the clitoris, and eventually coarse, masculine hair. It is particularly important to recognize the affected female during infancy so that correct assignment of sex can be made. Serious psychological disturbances accompany attempts to reverse sex in the older child.[12]

Male patients usually come to medical attention before they are 2 to 3 years old because of rapid growth, the early appearance of acne, excessive muscular development, and the premature appearance of secondary sex characteristics. The phallus may assume adult proportions, although the testes will remain infantile in size.

In about one-third of cases the 21-hydroxylase defect is complete causing an absolute deficiency of both cortisol and aldosterone. In these children it is extremely important to recognize the condition before a fatal salt-losing crisis supervenes. The early symptoms of salt loss may be overlooked in the affected male neonate because there has been no disturbance of normal male organogenesis and it is difficult, if not impossible, to perceive "overdevelopment" of the external genitalia at this age. Typically, the symptoms have their onset between the 6th and 14th day of life; there is loss of weight despite adequate fluid and food intake. The child goes on to vomit and to develop a profuse diarrhea leading to progressive dehydration, circulatory collapse and eventual cardiac arrest.

Treatment of the various congenital adrenogenital syndromes requires their early recognition and the life-long administration of appropriate suppressive doses of glucocorticoids and replacement doses of mineralocorticoid. Surgical aspects of therapy are concerned with the correction of external genitalia, which for the most part involves correction of the masculinized external organs in the female.

ADRENOCORTICAL CARCINOMA

The fully developed picture of masculinization in the adult female is seen rarely and is almost always indicative of an adrenocortical carcinoma. Affected individuals develop a masculine habitus with heavier musculature and loss of the feminine distribution of fat. A coarse growth of hair appears on the body and especially on the face, the temporal hairline recedes. The breasts atrophy, the voice deepens, and, paradoxically, there is an increase in heterosexual sex drive. An increasing tendency to amenorrhea is noted, the clitoris enlarges and a male escutcheon appears.

In the adult male, virilism does not attract attention. In almost all cases of virilizing tumors in males, the tumor has been discovered by chance.

Heinbecker et al.[48] in summarizing their experience with 83 cases of adrenocortical tumors, emphasized the fact that tumors of the adrenal cortex commonly produce a mixed pattern of hormonal secretion. Virilism of the female associated with manifestations of Cushing's syndrome strongly suggests adrenocortical carcinoma.

Rarely, adrenal carcinomas secrete estrogens which result in feminization.[30] In the male tender gynecomastia develops with penile atrophy and diminution in the size of the testes. Prepubertal females show signs of isosexual precocity with breast development, uterine bleeding, pubic and axillary hair, and advanced bone age.

Some adrenal carcinomas are either nonfunctioning or inefficiently synthesize steroid. By the time the patient has clinically recognizable virilization or Cushing's syndrome, the tumor will have attained such massive proportions that it displaces the kidney and may be palpable through the body wall.

LABORATORY INVESTIGATION OF VIRILISM

Urinary Steroid Excretion. Hypersecretion of adrenal androgens always results in an increased 17-KS excretion in the urine. Normally, prepubertal children excrete no more than 2 mg per 24 hours and children under 2 years of age much less. Children with congenital adrenal hyperplasia excrete from 3 to 40 mg of 17-KS in the urine per 24 hours. Adolescent and adult women normally excrete from 5 to 15 mg of 17-KS per 24 hours, whereas patients with virilizing hyperplasia of the adrenal cortex excrete from 16 to 80 mg per 24 hours. If the urinary 17-KS excretion is markedly elevated (in excess of 100 mg per day), the probability of adrenocortical carcinoma is high.[66]

When the urinary 17-KS are fractionated, dehydroepiandrosterone (DHA) is increased both in absolute and relative amounts, representing more than 50 percent of the total in the case of adrenal tumor. In virilizing hyperplasia of the adrenal cortex the level of DHA usually represents less than half the total 17-KS excretion in the urine.

In the common variety of congenital adrenal hyperplasia, patients produce an excess of the precursor 17-hydroxyprogesterone which is measurable in the plasma by radioimmunoassay methods, and excrete large amounts of its metabolite, pregnanetriol, in the urine (in excess of 4 mg per 24 hours). In the hypertensive type of congenital adrenal hyperplasia (11-hydroxylase deficiency), the plasma 11-deoxycortisol level is elevated.

Dexamethasone Suppression. Two milligrams of dexamethasone will suppress the 24 hour urinary excretion of 17-KS by at least 50 percent in virilizing hyperplasia of the adrenal cortex but there is no inhibition of excretion of this steroid in cases of adrenocortical tumor. This is the best single laboratory test to discriminate between hyperplasia and tumor.

ACTH Stimulation. The response of urinary 17-KS excretion to exogenous ACTH in cases of adrenocortical tumor is so variable that the test is of little value in differentiating these lesions from virilizing adrenal hyperplasia.[1]

Tumor Localization Studies. Intravenous pyelography and nephrotomography may reveal a tumor displacing the kidney. Heinbecker et al.[48] found that mottled calcification in the suprarenal area has often been associated with adrenal carcinoma.

When intravenous pyelography fails to reveal a tumor, selective adrenal arteriography is the most useful radiographic diagnostic procedure.[7]

Treatment of Adrenogenital Syndrome

The treatment of the adrenogenital syndrome is always medical except in rare cases of adrenal cortical tumor. It is directed first to the correction of adrenal insufficiency and second to the suppression of excessive release of ACTH. When it occurs, the adrenal insufficiency is clearly a more important factor and relates to the inability to synthesize cortisol and perhaps aldosterone. As indicated elsewhere, however, in most cases the excess release of ACTH allows for compensation of the enzymatic defect so that circulatory levels of the essential steroids is near normal but only at the expense of high levels of ACTH and thus of 17-ketosteroids with resultant virilization. In this syndrome levels of ACTH may be brought to normal by maintenance doses of cortisone. The progressive virilization will then cease and, to a degree, may reverse. If the patient has one of the salt-losing varieties of adrenogenital syndrome, 9α-fluorocortisol is also used. Therapy must be begun early in these children because the androgens will lead otherwise to early closure of the epiphyses and thus to dwarfism. With appropriate therapy, however, children will commonly attain nearly normal stature.

REFERENCES

1. Bartter, FC, Albright, F, Forbes, AP, Leaf, A, Dempsey, E, Carroll, E: The effects of adrenocorticotrophic hormone and cortisone in the adrenogenital syndrome associated with congenital adrenal hyperplasia:

an attempt to explain and correct its disordered hormonal pattern. J Clin Invest 30:237, 1951

2. Bartter, FC, Gann, DS: On the hemodynamic regulation of the secretion of aldosterone. Circulation 21:1016, 1960
3. Bartter, FC, Gann, DS, Thomas, JP: On the mechanisms of sodium retention in cardiac and hepatic disease, in Currie, AR, Symington, T, Grant JK: Human Adrenal Cortex. Baltimore, Williams & Wilkins, 1962
4. Bartter, FC, Mills, IH, Gann, DS: Increase in aldosterone secretion by carotid artery constriction in the dog and its prevention by thyrocarotid arterial junction denervation. J Clin Invest 39:1330, 1960
5. Bartter, FC, Mills, IH, Biglieri, EG, Delea, CS: Studies on the control and physiologic action of aldosterone. Recent Progr Hormone Res 15:311, 1959
6. Bartter, FC, Pronove, P., Gill, Jr., JR, MacCardle, RC: Hyperplasia of the juxtaglomerular complex with hyperaldosteronism and hypokalemic alkalosis. Am J Med 33:811, 1962
7. Bennet, AH, Harrison, JH, Thorn, GW: Neoplasms of the adrenal gland. J Urol 106:607, 1971
8. Besser, GM, Edwards, CRW: Cushing's syndrome. Clinics in Endocrinology and Metabolism 1:451, 1972
9. Biglieri, EG, Stockigt, JR, Schambelan, M: Adrenal mineralocorticoids causing hypertension. Am J Med 52:623, 1972
10. Blair-West, JR, Coghlan, JP, Denton, DS, Scoggins, BA, Wintour, EM, Wright, RD: Effect of change in sodium balance on the corticosteroid response to angiotein II. Aust J exp Biol med Sci 48:253, 1970
11. Bledsoe, T: Surgery and the adrenal cortex. Surg Clin N Amer 54:449, 1974
12. Bongiovanni, AM, Root, AW: The adrenogenital syndrome. NEJM 268:1283, 1342, 1391, 1963
13. Brown, JJ, Fraser, R, Lever, AF, Robertson, JIS: Aldosterone: Physiological and pathophysiological variations in man, in Clinics in Endocrinology and Metabolism, Saunders July, 1972
14. Bush, IE, Mahesh, VB: Adrenocortical hyperfunction with sudden onset of hirsutism. J Endocrinol 18:1, 1959
15. Conn, JW, Bookstein, JJ, Cohen, EL: Renin-secreting juxtaglomerular-cell adenoma. Preoperative clinical and angiographic diagnosis. Radiology 106:543, 1973
16. Conn, JW, Knopf, RF, Nesbit, RM: Clinical characteristics of primary aldosteronism from analysis of 145 cases. Am J Surg 107:159, 1964
17. Conn, JW, Morita, R, Cohen, EL, Beierwaltes, WH, McDonald, WJ, Herwig, KR: Primary aldosteronism. Photoscanning of tumors after administration of 131I-19-Iodocholesterol. Arch Int Med 129:417, 1972
18. Conn, JW, Rovner, DR, Cohen, EC, Bookstein, JJ, Cerny, JC, Lucas, CP: Preoperative diagnosis of primary aldosteronism. Arch Int Med 123:113, 1969

19. Cryer, GL, Gann, DS: Location of vagal receptors controlling adrenal corticosteroid secretion. Am J Physiol 225:1346, 1973
20. Cushing, H: The basophil adenomas of the pituitary body and their clinical manifestations (pituitary basophilism) Bull Johns Hopkins Hosp 1:137, 1932
21. Dallman, MF, Jones, MT: Corticosteroid feedback control of stress-induced ACTH secretion in Brain-Pituitary-Adrenal Interrelationships, Basel Karger, 1973, p 176
22. Dallman, MF, Yates, FE: Dynamic asymmetries in the corticosteroid feedback path and distribution-metabolism-binding elements of the adrenocortical system. Ann NY Acad Sci 156:696, 1969
23. Davis, JO: The regulation of aldosterone secretion in A.B. Eisenstein (ed) The Adrenal Cortex, Boston, Little, Brown 1968, p. 203
24. Davis, WW, Burwell, LR, Casper, AGT, Bartter, FC: Sites of action of sodium depletion on aldosterone biosynthesis in the dog. J Clin Invest 47:1425, 1968
25. Dawson, DB, Dingman JF: Hazards of proton-beam pituitary irradiation. NEJM 282:1434, 1970
26. Egdahl, RH: Pituitary-adrenal response following trauma to the isolated leg. Surgery 46:9, 1959
27. Egdahl, RH: Surgery of the adrenal gland. NEJM 278:939, 1968
28. Egdahl, RH, Kahn, PC, Melby, JC: Unilateral adrenalectomy for aldosteronomas localized preoperatively by differential adrenal vein catheterization. Surgery 64:117, 1968
29. Egdahl, RH, Kahn, PC, Melby, JC: Role of angiography in surgery of the adrenal. Am J Surg 117:480, 1969
30. Gabrilove, JL, Sharma, DC, Wotiz, HH, Dorfman, RI: Feminizing adrenocortical tumors in male: review of 52 cases including case report. Medicine 44:37, 1965
31. Gann, DS: Carotid vascular receptors and control of adrenal corticosteroid secretion. Am J Physiol 211:193, 1966
32. Gann, DS: Parameters of the stimulus initiating the adrenocortical response to hemorrhage. Ann NY Acad Sci 156:740, 1969
33. Gann, DS: The control of adrenal secretion of cortisol in Brown, JHU, Gann, DS (eds), Engineering Principles in Physiology. NY, Academic Press 1973, vol 1, p. 213
34. Gann, DS, Cryer GL: Models of adrenal cortical control. Adv Biomed Engr 2:1, 1972
35. Gann, DS, Cryer GL: Feedback control of ACTH secretion by cortisol in Brodish, A, Redgate ES, (ed), Brain-Pituitary-Adrenal Interrelationships. Basel, Karger, 1973, p. 197
36. Gann, DS, Cryer, GL: ACTH changes after sequential hemorrhage in the presence and absence of cortisol. Proc 56th Mtg Endocrine Soc, Endocrinol 94:A-239, 1974
37. Gann, DS, Egdahl, RH: Responses of adrenal corticosteroid secretion to hypotension and hypovolemia. J Clin Invest 44:1, 1965

38. Gann, DS, Travis, RH: Mechanisms of hemodynamics control of secretion of aldosterone in the dog. Am J Physiol 207:1095, 1964
39. Gann, DS, Wright, HK: Effects of trauma on sodium metabolism and urinary concentrating ability. J Surg Research 6:93, 1966
40. Gann, DS, Delea, CS, Gill Jr., JR, Thomas, JP, Bartter, FC: Control of aldosterone secretion by change of body potassium in normal man. Am J Physiol 207:104, 1964
41. Gibbs, FP: Central nervous system lesions that block release of ACTH caused by traumatic stress. Am J Physiol 217:78, 1969
42. Gifford, S, Gunderson, JG: Cushing's disease as a psychosomatic disorder. Perspect Biol Med 13:169, 1970
43. Grizzle, WE, Dallman, MF, Schramm, LP, Gann, DS: Inhibitory facilitatory hypothalamic areas mediating and ACTH release in the cat. Endocrinol, 95:1450, 1974
44. Grizzle, WE, Johnson, RN, Schramm, LP, Gann, DS: Hypothalamic cells in an area mediating ACTH release respond to right atrial stretch. AM J Physiol, in press
45. Harris, GW: Neural Control of the Pituitary Gland. London, Edward Arnold, 1955
46. Hedge, GA, Smelik, PG: Corticotropin release: inhibition by intrahypothalamic implantation of atropine. Science 159:891, 1968
47. Hedge, GA, Yates, MB, Marcus, R, Yates, FE: Site of action of vasopressin in causing corticotropin release. Endocrinology 79:328, 1966
48. Heinbecker, P, O'Neal, LW, Ackerman, LV: Functioning and nonfunctioning adrenal cortical tumors. Surg Gynec Obst 105:21, 1957
49. Hellman, L, Weitzman, ED, Roffwarg, H, Fukushima, DK, Yoshida, K, Gallagher, TF: Cortisol is secreted episodically in Cushing's syndrome. J Clin Endocrinol Metab 30:686, 1970
50. Herman, AH, Mack, E, Egdahl, RH: The relationship of adrenal perfusion to corticosteroid secretion in prolonged hemorrhagic shock. Surg Gynecol Obstet 132:795, 1971
51. Hiroshige, T: CRF assay by intrapituitary injection through the parapharyngeal approach and its physiological validation, in Brain-Pituitary-Adrenal Interrelationships. Basel, Karger, 1973, p 57
52. Hodge, RL, Lowe, RD, Vane, JR: The effects of alteration of blood-volume on the concentration of circulating angiotensin in anesthetized dogs. J Physiol 185:613, 1966
53. Hodge, RL, Lowe, RD, Vane, JR: Increased angiotensin formation in response to carotid occlusion in the dog. Nature 211:491, 1966
54. Hume, DM: The method of hypothalamic regulation of pituitary and adrenal secretion in response to trauma, in S. B. Curri, Martini, L, (ed), Pathophysiologia, Diencephalica, Wein, Springer-Verlag 1958, p 217
55. Hutter, AM, Jr., Kayhoe, DE: Adrenal Cortical Carcinoma. Am J Med 41:572, 1966

56. Kahn, PC: The radiologic identification of functioning adrenal tumors. Radiol Clin North Am 5:221, 1967
57. Kahn, PC, Kelleher, MD, Egdahl, RH, Melby, JC: Adrenal arteriography and venography in primary aldosteronism. Radiology 101:71, 1971
58. Kaplan NM, Bartter, FC: The effect of ACTH, renin, angiotensin II and various precursors on biosynthesis of aldosterone by adrenal slices. J Clin Invest 41:715, 1962
59. Laragh, JH: Renal and adrenal factors in hypertension: diagnostic approaches. Bull NY Acad Med 45:859, 1969
60. Laragh, JH, Stoerk, HC: On the mechanism of secretion of the sodium-retaining hormone (aldosterone) within the body. J Clin Invest 34:913, 1955
61. Laragh, JH, Sealey, JE, Sommers, SC: Patterns of adrenal secretion and urinary excretion of aldosterone and plasma renin activity in normal and hypertensive subjects. Circ Res 18, suppl 1:58, 1966.
62. Lieberman, LM, Beierwaltes, WH, Conn, JW, Ansari, AN, Nishiyama, H: Diagnosis of adrenal disease by visualization of human adrenal glands with 131I-19-iodocholesterol. NEJM 285:1387, 1971
63. McCormick, JR, Herman, AH, Lien, WM, Egdahl, RH: Hydrocortisone metabolism in the adrenalectomized dog: the quantitative significance of each organ system in the total metabolic clearance of hydrocortisone. Endocrinology 94:17, 1974
64. Melby, JC: personal communication
65. Melby, JC: Primary aldosteronism, Practitioner 200:519, 1968
66. Melby, JC: Assessment of adrenocortical function. NEJM 285:735. 1971
67. Melby, JC: Case records of the Massachusetts General Hospital. Case 39-1972, NEJM 287:656, 1972
68. Melby, JC, Spark, RF, Dale, SL, Egdahl, RH, Kahn, PC: Diagnosis and localization of aldosterone-producing adenomas by adrenal vein catheterization. NEJM 277:1050, 1967
69. Messerli, FH, et al. Mineralocorticoid secretion in low renin benign essential hypertension. Proc 56th Mtg Endocrine Soc, Endocrinol 94:A-63, 1974
70. Mills, IH, Brooks, RV, Prunty, FTG: The relationship between the production of cortisol and of androgen by the human adrenal cortex, in Human Adrenal Cortex, op. cit. (3), p. 204
71. Mobley, JE, Headstream, JW, Melby, JC: Primary aldosteronism: preoperative preparation with spironolactone. JAMA 180:1056, 1962
72. Muller, AF, Manning, EL, Riondel, AM: Diurnal variation of aldosterone related to position and activity in normal subjects and patients with pituitary insufficiency, in *An International* Symposium on Aldosterone A. F. Muller and C. M. O'Connor (ed), Boston, Little, Brown 1958, p. 111

73. Nelson, DH, Meakin, JW, Thorn, GW: ACTH producing pituitary tumors following adrenalectomy for Cushing's syndrome. Am Int Med 52:560, 1960
74. Ng, KKF, Vane, JR: Fate of angiotensin I in the circulation. Nature 218:144, 1968
75. Orth, DN, Liddle, GW: Results of treatment in 108 patients with Cushing's syndrome. NEJM 285:243, 1971
76. Ohsawa, N: Effect of administration of ACTH on adrenal responsiveness of hypophysectomized rats. Endocrinology 77:461, 1965
77. Redgate, ES: Spinal cord and ACTH release in adrenalectomized rats following electrical stimulation. Endocrinology 70:263, 1962
78. Scott, HW, Jr, Liddle, GW, Harris, AP, Foster, JH: Diagnosis and treatment of Cushing's syndrome. Ann Surg 155:696, 1962
79. St Cyr, MJ, Sancho, JM, Melby, JC: Quantitation of plasma aldosterone by radioimmunoassay. Clin Chem 18:1395, 1972
80. Thorn, GW, Lauler, DP: Clinical therapeutics of adrenal disorders. Am J Med 53:673, 1972
81. Tyler, FH, West, CD: Laboratory evaluation of disorders of the adrenal cortex. Am J Med 53:664, 1972
82. Urquhart, J: Adrenal blood flow and the adrenocortical response to corticotropin. Am J Physiol 209:1162, 1965
83. Williams, RH: Textbook of Endocrinology, Philadelphia, Saunders, 1968, p. 1143
84. Vander, AJ: Control of renin release. Physiol Rev 47:359, 1967
85. Williams, RH: op. cit. (83) p. 317
86. Yates, FE, Russell, SM, Dallman, MF, Hedge, GA, McCann, SM, Dhariwal, APS: Potentiation by vasopressin of corticotropin release induced by corticotropin-releasing factor. Endocrinology 83:3, 1971
87. Yates, FE, Maran, JW, Cryer, GL, Gann, DS: The pituitary adrenal cortical system: stimulation and inhibition of secretion of corticotropin. MTP International Review of Science S.M. McCann (ed) London, Butterworth 1974, Ch 4
88. Zimmerman, G, Casey, JH, Block, HS, Bickel, EY, Covrik, K: Excretion of aldosterone by the postoperative patient, Surg Forum 6:3, 1956

3

The Adrenal Medulla

BIOSYNTHESIS OF CATECHOLAMINES

The stepwise transformation of tyrosine into epinephrine (adrenaline) seemed logical to thoughtful chemists as early as 1910. Casimir Funk,[38] a respected scientist of the time, commented that, "the question of the formation of adrenaline in the animal body has engaged much attention. The two amino acids that suggest themselves as parent substances are obviously tyrosine and phenylalanine . . . It may well be, however, that the formation of adrenaline takes place in several steps and that different tissues of the body are necessary."

Thirty years later H. C. Blashko,[9,10] not long after his return to England from Professor Walter Cannon's laboratory at Harvard, took up the question of the biosynthesis of adrenaline (Fig. 3-1) and in 1939, with remarkable prescience, suggested that the steps involved in the biosynthesis of epinephrine were as follows: the 3-hydroxylation of tyrosine to form dihydroxyphenylalanine (dopa).

The decarboxylation of dopa formed 3,4-dihydroxyphenylethylamine (dopamine); then dopamine in Blashko's scheme was hydroxylated on the beta carbon of the side chain to form 3,4-dihydroxyphenylalpha-amino; beta-ethanol, which we know as norepinephrine.

Norepinephrine was the logical precursor of epinephrine. Subsequently referred to as "Blashko's Hypothesis," investigations of the next 20 years verified each step he predicted. By now the enzymes involved in each step of this biosynthesis have been identified and important features of their activity described.

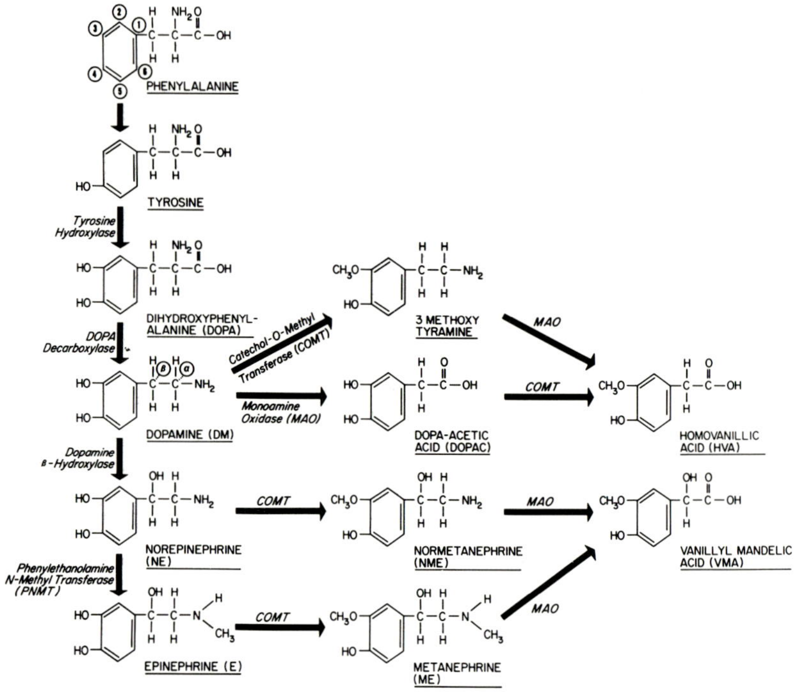

Fig. 3-1. Biosynthesis and major metabolic pathways of the catecholamines.

In 1946, U.S. von Euler,[26] Professor of Physiology at the Karolinska Institute in Stockholm, fitted in the last piece of Blashko's puzzle by demonstrating for the first time the presence of endogenous norepinephrine (noradrenaline) in adrenergic nerves. The discovery of endogenous adrenal norepinephrine was announced simultaneously by Peter Holtz, a pharmacologist in Frankfurt.

Soon after discovering endogenous norepinephrine, von Euler[27,28] pointed out that norepinephrine reproduced faithfully all the biological actions of Cannon's Sympathin-E, a circulating factor of unknown structure with profound cardiovascular effects. Thus, norepinephrine emerged in the late 1940s as a compound native to animal tissue with two distinct roles; one as a precursor of epinephrine and the other as a biologically active neurally released hormone with important effects on the circulation and metabolism.

Important insights into the termination of action of the catecholamines coincided with, and developed from, these discoveries. While it had been appreciated for years that biogenic amines were oxidatively deaminated in the body, this action occurred too slowly to account for the brisk disappearance of intravenously injected norepinephrine or epinephrine, the half-life of which was 3 minutes or less.[7] Other methods of termination such as glucuronide binding, acid hydrolyzable binding, and free excretion all could be demonstrated; the fractions of injected amines involved in these mechanisms were disappointingly small and could not account for the largest portion of injected amines.

In 1957, Julius Axelrod[4,5] of the National Institutes of Health demonstrated that the addition of a methoxy (CH_3–O–) linkage on the 3 position of the phenyl ring occurred biologically under favorable circumstances (Fig. 3-1), the chief one of which was the presence of a suitable methyl group donor such as *S*-adenosyl-methionine. Thus, epinephrines conversion to metanephrine was soon established as was the comparable O-methylation for norepinephrine which formed normetanephrine. Axelrod called the enzyme catechol, 3-*O*-methyl transferase. These metanephrine compounds are clinically important and are identifiable in urine and other body fluids and tissues.

In 1959, Axelrod and his co-workers demonstrated that small quantities of radioactively labeled epinephrine were, following their intravenous injection into cats, taken up from the circulation and stored in adrenergically innervated tissues.[6] Prior to this it was appreciated that significant fractions of large quantities of injected catecholamines were taken up into tissues such as the heart and spleen. This uptake was into neuronal storage pools from which the catecholamines could subsequently be released by appropriate reflex stimulation and post ganglionic adrenergic nerve depolarization. It was soon apparent that tissue uptake of circulating catecholamines was an important mechanism for terminating the action of circulating catecholamines. More recently, the kinetics of the uptake process for the catecholamines have been studied in depth by Leslie Iversen at Cambridge University.[67,68]

With these and numerous other facts available, it is now possible to form a dynamic picture of catecholamine synthesis and release which follows this general pattern. The biosynthesis of norepinephrine and epinephrine takes place in postganglionic adrenergic neurons, the formation of dopa and dopamine taking place in the cytoplasm of the axonal cell. Dopamine then enters the catecholamine storage vesicle near the nerve terminal where its conversion to noradrenaline by the enzyme dopamine-beta-hydroxylase takes place. Only in the storage vesicles of the chromaffin cells of the adrenal medulla is it possible for appreciable quantities of norepinephrine to be converted to epinephrine. The enzyme responsible is phenyl-ethanolamine-*N*-methyl-transferase (PNMT). For this action PNMT is known to require a large quantity of cortisol.[98]

This is delivered to the adrenal medulla by an adrenal portal venous system described by Flint in 1911.[33]

Once stored in the neuronal vesicles, the catecholamines dopamine and norepinephrine, are in close proximity to the ending of the sympathetic nerve from which the depolarization associated with a nerve impulse will trigger the exocytosis which releases these catecholamines into the synaptic cleft and into the circulation. Two things happen when these catecholamines are released. First, as many as 25,000 effector cells may respond to the discharge of one postganglionic adrenergic neuron; second, the catecholamines released into the general circulation can then reach adrenergic receptor sites on other effector organs through the general circulation into which they are released.[7] The catecholamines are then terminated by any of the previously mentioned means particularly uptake into storage vesicles of adrenergic nerves, and/or metabolism by specific enzymes in the circulation, i.e., catechol-*O*-methyl-transferase or metabolism in tissues of the body, amine-oxidase as well as catechol-*O*-methyl-transferase.

Increased activity of adrenergic neurons causes an increase in the biosynthesis of norepinephrine from tyrosine. The enzyme tyrosine hydroxylase in turn is inhibited by excessive catecholamines and thus tissue levels of dopa, dopamine and norepinephrine may remain remarkably constant in the face of greatly increased adrenergic neuronal activity and catecholamine turnover. Studies with radioactively labeled catecholamines are necessary to describe the catecholamine turnover rate accurately.

The 3 to 6 percent of catecholamines excreted free in the urine can easily be measured by highly sensitive specific fluorometric, or more recently by enzymatic techniques especially designed for the catecholamines. Approximately 110 μg of dopamine, 20 μg of norepinephrine, and 5 μg of epinephrine are normally excreted free in the urine of resting adult subjects each day. Glucuronides and acid hydrolyzable linkages account for a roughly equal quantity but it is laborious to measure these.

Epinephrine, formed in the adrenal medulla and released into the circulation from its chromaffin cells, is taken up by adrenergically innervated tissue in general and can stimulate adrenergic receptors on the surface of effector cells.

Acetylcholine is a potent stimulus of epinephrine and norepinephrine release from the innervated adrenal gland. This is not surprising since depolarization of the preganglionic and postganglionic sympathetic fibers is a cholinergically driven event and capable of as finely graded and discriminant action as any other cholinergic motor system. Professor

J. H. Burn and his colleagues at Oxford have repeatedly reemphasized this point and are largely responsible for promulgating the view that it is inaccurate to speak of an adrenergic nervous system as such.[13,14,15] It is more accurately descriptive to think of adrenergic effector units of cholinergically stimulated pre- and postganglionic neurons. The exception to this is in the adrenal medulla whose catecholamine containing chromaffin cells are, in fact, postganglionic being innervated by the terminal dendrites of preganglionic nerve fibers. Precisely how many adrenal chromaffin cells are innervated by a given preganglionic neuron has never been studied and it would be of interest to know if this innervation is more discrete, that is, fewer chromaffin cells per preganglionic neuron than is the case for postganglionic adrenergic fibers.

The adrenal medulla is recognized, on the basis of histochemical studies of Hillarp[63] and subsequently from immunofluorescent studies of Fuxe et al, to have islands of cells that contain norepinephrine and other, more frequently occurring cells containing both norepinephrine and epinephrine. In both groups of cells dopamine beta-hydroxylase can be demonstrated but only the epinephrine containing cells contain PNMT.[64,65]

There is evidence from hypothalamic stimulation studies of Folkow and von Euler that these islands of cells are discretely innervated and may be selectively stimulated.[29] Stimulation of some hypothalamic loci caused the release of a mixture of epinephrine and norepinephrine into adrenal vein blood and stimulation of other loci pure norepinephrine or pure epinephrine release.

The only organ incapable of taking up catecholamines from the circulation is the brain. The catecholamines do not cross the so-called blood–brain barrier and hence dopamine and norepinephrine, widely distributed in the brain and of particular importance in regulating fine motor activity, are synthesized in the neurons of the brain in a manner similar to that for peripheral adrenergic nerves.[6] Small quantities of epinephrine are synthesized in the brain by functionally important "epinephrinergic" neurons. The PNMT involved can be identified by immunofluorescent techniques and probably differs somewhat from adrenal PNMT. Glucuronide binding of catecholamines is felt to be more important as a mechanism of termination of catecholamine activity in the central nervous system than it is in other tissues.[88]

Tyrosine hydroxylase, dopamine hydroxylase, and PNMT are all reduced by hypophysectomy. Administration of ACTH will restore the normal activity of all three of these enzymes in hypophysectomized animals.[5,6]

PHYSIOLOGICAL RELEASE OF CATECHOLAMINES

The most sensitive and abundant data on reflex stimulation of catecholamine release concerns the adrenal gland. There are several reasons for this, the most obvious being that the total adrenal venous effluent can be easily diverted into the adrenal vein. This vein can be selectively cannulated in many animal species; the sampling time from the adrenal cannula will give an accurate estimation of adrenal blood flow. Division of the splanchnic nerve just superior to the adrenal gland almost completely abolishes the epinephrine and norepinephrine secretory response of the adrenal gland to reflex stimulation without influencing the adrenal blood flow. Of further significance for critical study is that the content of epinephrine and norepinephrine in adrenal vein blood is sufficiently high to permit the repeated measurement of these catecholamines on serial blood samples taken under well-defined experimental conditions. If arterial catecholamines are measured simultaneously, it is possible to derive authentic adrenal secretion rates for epinephrine and norepinephrine in a wide variety of experimental laboratory conditions. No other endocrine organ is arranged so conveniently for laboratory investigation.

Experimental Resting Conditions

Normal, trained, conscious dogs have an epinephrine content of roughly 0.2 μg per liter and norepinephrine 0.2 μg per liter in systemic venous blood. Experimentally in healthy dogs under sodium pentobarbital anesthesia, plasma epinephrine levels abruptly rise, approximately 10 fold, to values of roughly 2 μg per liter while norepinephrine levels are unchanged.[48]

If anesthetized dogs are permitted to breath room air either on their own or have air delivered by volume respirator, the secretion rate of epinephrine from the innervated adrenal gland is sustained at about 0.3 μg per minute. If 98 percent oxygen and 2 percent CO_2 is breathed spontaneously through an endotracheal tube by the anesthetized dog, the respiratory rate slows to 2 or 3 respirations per minute and adrenal epinephrine secretion rates rise progressively to 0.75 μg per minute through a 3 hour experiment. If one delivers a gas mixture of 98 percent O_2 and 2 CO_2 by volume respirator, thereby minimizing chemoreceptor activity, the adrenal release of epinephrine and norepinephrine is minimized to 0.1 μg per minute or less and continues so throughout the course of a 3 hour experiment. During this time arterial pH and pCO_2 remain in a physiological range.[49]

Experimental Reflex Stimulation of Catecholamine Release

ACUTE HYPOVOLEMIA

Acute hypovolemia to 50 mm Hg mean arterial pressure (about one-quarter the estimated blood volume) will excite the adrenal release of epinephrine and norepinephrine in the dog anesthetized with pentobarbital, raising the secretion rate of epinephrine as high as 2.1 μg per minute 60 minutes following hemorrhage. Splanchnic nerve section completely abolishes this response[56] but does not deplete adrenal catecholamines.[86]

The volume of blood shed to achieve 50 mm Hg mean arterial pressure is remarkably constant, about 26 ml per kg body weight. The one exception to this is in animals with acute adrenalectomy. Adrenalectomy animals are uniquely sensitive to volume contraction and become markedly hypotensive to volume losses of as little as 7 to 10 ml blood loss per kg body weight.

OTHER CARDIOVASCULAR REFLEXES

One basic question raised by the secretory response to acute hypovolemia is whether it is blood volume contraction that stimulates reflex epinephrine release or a decrease in arterial blood pressure that does so. There is some insight into this question. Adreno-femoral shunts were placed in dogs in which bilateral innervated isolated carotid sinus loops had been prepared. In normal dogs, an increase in the carotid sinus pressure caused a compensatory decrease in mean systemic arterial pressure to less than 50 mm Hg. No secretory inhibition from the adrenal gland was associated with this nor was there a secretory burst when the isolated carotid sinus pressure was lowered causing a rise in mean systemic arterial pressure. Finally, if one contracts the blood volume by bleeding the same animals acutely to 50 mm Hg (mean arterial pressure), the typical adrenal secretory burst occurs regardless of what pressure is perfusing the isolated carotid sinuses.[54]

A number of considerations are raised by these observations.[54] First of all, the systemic pressure adjustment from the carotid sinus is, as shown by M. de Burgh Daly and his associates,[2] an adrenergically mediated phenomenon in that it can be prevented with alpha adrenergic receptor blockade by phenoxybenzamine. It is also known that epinephrine release can be stimulated by carotid sinus preparations if pulsatile wave forms in a critical range of mean pressure and pulse amplitude are brought to the sinus preparations.[54] Furthermore, prolongation of the time to achieve maximum arterial pressure, $\Delta p/\Delta t$, does appear to increase, moderately, adrenal epinephrine release.

A principle emerging from these sets of observations is that adrenergically mediated resistance changes (and hence blood pressure regulation) are not always accompanied by the separate adrenergic phenomenon of epinephrine release. Thus, while the adrenergic nervous system is capable of total responsiveness as in the fright and flight responses described by Cannon, it is also capable of finely graded discriminate activity in which only certain adrenergic effector systems are active. Physiologically these responses appear to represent an appropriate reaction to the stimulus in question.

METABOLIC STIMULI

Hypoglycemia. Cannon[17] appreciated that lowering the blood sugar below 40 mg per 100 ml blood excited the release of adrenal epinephrine and that this was a reflex effect prevented by prior section of the adrenal splanchnic nerve. The release of epinephrine was considered to be purposeful ("homeostatic" to use Cannon's term) in that the released epinephrine stimulated the breakdown of glycogen into sugar and helped raise blood glucose to physiological levels.

The hypoglycemic effect on epinephrine release was studied in depth by Duner[23] who first of all confirmed Cannon's observations of the epinephrine secretory response to hypoglycemia and abolition of this response by section of the splanchnic nerve. Also Duner reduced adrenal epinephrine release in animals by microinjections of glucose solution into the hypothalamus. Microinjections of saline did not produce the same effect. Cross circulation to the head from a hyperglycemic dog had the same inhibitory effect on adrenal epinephrine release.

Hypoxia. Hypoxia is often considered a uniquely potent stimulant of adrenal catecholamine release. To a large degree this conviction is based on experiments performed a long time ago in which violent measures were tested such as asphyxia from tracheal clamping for 30 seconds or inhalation of 100 percent nitrogen for 30 seconds.

When dogs under pentobarbital anesthesia inhale 10 percent O_2, 90 percent nitrogen through an endotracheal tube there is, after 2 hours, a substantial increase in the adrenal secretion rate of epinephrine to 7 μg per minute. In the first 2 hours of this hypoxia, less striking increases, 1 μg per minute, in epinephrine release occur. The arterial pO_2 of the animals breathing 10 percent O_2 was consistently around 30 mm Hg, representing a definite but not profound hypoxia. Arterial pH during this hypoxia was between 7.2 and 7.3. This secretory response to hypoxia can be prevented by prior splanchnic nerve section.

Cold. Decreased body temperature, probably sensed by temperature sensitive cells in the hypothalamus, will elicit an increase in catecholamine release. The biological oxidation stimulated by the catecholamines help provide that heat energy needed to restore body temperature to normal. The phenomenon has been studied in depth by several workers. One can refer to the excellent study of LeDuc[73] for more detail.

HORMONAL EFFECTS ON REFLEX CATECHOLAMINE RELEASE

Certain hormones are thought to influence the magnitude of reflex catecholamine release. A great deal of this literature is fuzzy and it is difficult to be certain of the significance of, for example, the effects of adrenal steroids or thyroid hormones on catecholamine release. It is clear that hypothyroidism is associated with elevated circulating norepinephrine levels and accentuated reflex norepinephrine release.[18] This increase may be related to decreased metabolism of norepinephrine in hypothyroidism rather than to increased norepinephrine release.[90] Mornex has evidence indicating exaggerated epinephrine release in response to hypoglycemia in hyperthyroidism.[78] In a small series of cases we found contrary results as did Leak in cases he studied.[44,71] The possibility of increased catecholamine turnover in hyperthyroidism should be studied in depth.[46]

Angiotensin II, in recent studies, appears to have a fundamental permissive effect on reflex catecholamine release.[55]

Emotional Stimuli of Catecholamine Release

It was clear to Cannon and other early students that fright was a potent stimulus for catecholamine release. This was considered important to the poised psychic arousal initiated by fright.

Sophisticated insights into mental activity and related urinary catecholamine excretion have validated Cannon's general concept of the importance of the central nervous system in the selective stimulation of epinephrine release. We have already mentioned the hypothalamic stimulation studies of Folkow and U.S. von Euler.[34]

Following adrenal medullectomy executive monkeys, i.e., monkeys engaged in chronic avoidance of electrical shock by the successful use of a telegraph key, tend to consistently excrete more free norepinephrine in the urine than control monkeys with adrenal medullectomy in the identical environment.[59]

There is available still more sensitive evidence of central nervous system involvement in catecholamine release. Sleeping subjects excrete less catecholamine than awake subjects. Frankenhauser,[35] in a provocative study from the Karolinska Institute, studied free urinary epinephrine and norepinephrine excretion in normal Swedish high school students. The students were seated comfortably in a classroom and were given problem solving exercises for 90 minutes. Subjects with high excretion rates of both hormones tended to perform better in the entire stress session than subjects with low excretion rates. High excretion rates of both hormones tended to be associated with a decrease in emotional intensity to the testing situation.

Direct Glandular Stimulation of Catecholamine Release

Low pH blood perfusing the adrenal will stimulate the release of epinephrine and norepinephrine. This also holds true for the release of norepinephrine from peripheral storage sites. As shown by Morris and Millar[77] and others, this pH effect becomes marked as the pH of the perfusing blood falls below 6.8. Spontaneous breathing of a 30 percent carbon dioxide, 70 percent oxygen, gas mixture by anesthetized dogs stimulates a violent catecholamine secretory response from the adrenal. In this situation, epinephrine secretion rates as high as 40 μg per minute are found. This is the highest release rate we have seen in the dog and it occurs within an hour of introduction of the 30 percent CO_2 mixture. This secretory rate exceeds by about 10 fold the maximal release achieved by the most potent reflex stimulation. This response to hypercarbia can be prevented by infusion of an efficient buffer which maintains the arterial pH at physiological levels. The release can also be prevented by mechanical delivery of the same gas mixture which maintains arterial pH at 6.9 to 7.0.[48]

Ionized calcium stimulates the release of adrenal catecholamines and probably peripherally stored amines as well. Calcium is thought to make the vesicular membrane of storage granules permeable to catecholamines and other molecules in the cytoplasm.

Whether there is a group of adrenal catecholamine release stimuli that act directly on chromaffin cells, but only act if the glandular innervation maintains a constant tonic activity, is a question of interest for which no answer is currently available. Detailed neurophysiologic impulse analysis and concomitant catecholamine secretion rates in the splanchnic nerve and the chromaffin cells would be necessary to evaluate this point. The denervated adrenal medulla, even though its synthesis of catecholamines and levels of stored catecholamines are maintained at the level of the innervated gland[86] is thought to respond to few physiologically active stimuli.

Pharmacologic Stimulation of Catecholamine Release

It is impossible to describe here the mechanisms of action of the large groups and varieties of drugs stimulating catecholamine release both from the adrenal gland and adrenergic nerves in general. A few agents are of sufficient interest to mention.

A large variety of sympathomimetic and some sympatholytic drugs stimulate adrenal and peripheral catecholamine release. For example, reserpine and guanethidine stimulate the acute release of epinephrine and norepinephrine at the initial administration. In addition to this action, these drugs block adrenergic transmission between the termination of the postganglionic neuron and the effector cell. These two drugs are best known for their action of chronically depleting tissue levels of epinephrine and norepinephrine throughout the body including the central nervous system. Certain drugs which act on tissue stores of catecholamine, tyramine for example, are felt to cause release by displacing catecholamines from a labile neuronal pool.

Alpha adrenergic receptor blockade as, for example, with phenoxybenzamine (dibenzyline) or with shorter acting phentolamine (Regitine®) is associated with acutely increased circulating catecholamine levels. Two factors probably contribute to this increase; one is that re-uptake of circulating catecholamines into neuronal storage pools is also blocked by phenoxybenzamine. There is probably also increased pre- and postganglionic neural activity elicited by phenoxybenzamine since with the sympathetic ganglionic blockade conferred by spinal anesthesia, this rise in circulating norepinephrine and epinephrine following alpha adrenergic receptor blockade is prevented.

We hope these few remarks concerning the wide variety of stimuli influencing neuronally mediated and neuronally independent catecholamine release will create an awareness of the complexity of events represented in a simple expression of plasma levels and free excretion rates of catecholamines and their metabolites. The determination of these excretion rates and plasma levels forms the keystone for clinical evaluation of the autonomic nervous system in clinical medicine.

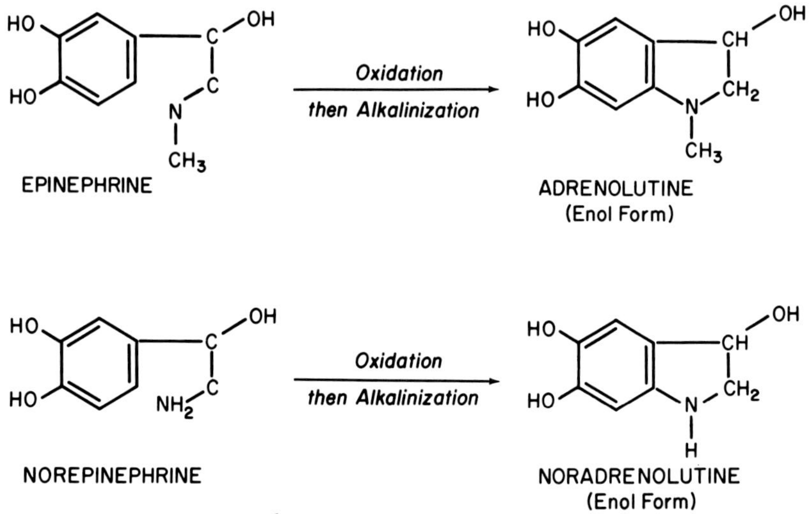

Fig. 3-2. Depicted is the oxidation of catecholamines involved in the formation of the highly fluorogenic tri-hydroxy-indole (THI) derivatives. These compounds are used in fluorimetric catecholamine analysis.

Because these measurements are so fundamental, some insight into the commonly used analytical techniques is helpful.

CATECHOLAMINE ANALYSIS

The fluorometric trihydroxyindole analytical technique for urinary epinephrine and norepinephrine, more exacting than many clinical laboratory procedures, can nevertheless, be mastered by a competent laboratory technologist. The fluorometric determination of oxidized products of the metanephrines, probably also as hydroxyindole derivatives, is more exacting and error prone because it requires a sophisticated grasp of column chromatography with Amberlite. Thus it is not uncommon to find figures for normal metanephrine and normetanephrine excretion somewhat lower than those originally published by Taniguchi et al.[95] It is, therefore, essential to know what normal ranges are for the laboratory reporting metanephrine results. The metanephrines are usually measured both as free and acid hydrolyzable metabolites and expressed as the sum of these two.

Vanillylmandelic acid (VMA) the end product of oxidative deamination and 3-*O*-methylation of norepinephrine and epinephrine, is normally excreted in the urine at a rate of 6 to 8 mg per day, 200 to 400 fold greater quantities than those of free, unbound epinephrine and norepinephrine. The colorimetric reaction used for VMA determination is crude and unless chromatographic separation of VMA from the sulfates in the urine is made, the VMA determination is flagrantly inaccurate.

Measurement of urinary dopamine excretion is now feasible as is the determination of dopamine metabolites such as dihydroxyphenylacetic acid (DOPAC), homovanillic acid, and others. All the catecholamine metabolites can be measured critically if proper attention to analytical detail is maintained. In measuring the less commonly determined catecholamines and metabolites, it is important to establish the identity of the compound by first confirming that the fluorescence activating and emission spectra of the sample are identical to those of an authentic sample of the compound in question.

Measurement of blood plasma concentration of epinephrine and norepinephrine in the physiological range of 0.15 μg per liter epinephrine and 0.20 μg per liter norepinephrine is notoriously capricious with the trihydroxyindole technique. If large blood samples, 30 to 40 ml are drawn, sufficient catecholamine is available, 6 to 8 ng, for reasonable accuracy with the trihydroxyindole determination of each of these catecholamines. At these low quantities of catecholamine, i.e., less than 10 ng, the standard trihydroxyindole curve is not linear and furthermore, is not the same for any two different analytical runs. Thus, for plasma determination with the trihydroxyindole technique a standard curve must be determined for each analytical run used; the standard quantities of catecholamines used for the standard curve must embrace the actual quantities of catecholamine being measured. At least 75 percent recovery of internal and external standards must be achieved. Using such admittedly rigorous techniques, reasonably accurate results can be obtained for plasma samples in the high physiologic range.

More recently a double isotopic technique using conversion of epinephrine and norepinephrine to their metanephrine metabolites has been described by Engelman and Portnoy.[25] The technique is not without its problems; nevertheless, it has the important advantage of linearity of the curve down to 1 ng of catecholamine and requires only 10 ml of blood.

An ideal in plasma analysis of epinephrine and norepinephrine is a technique permitting the constant monitoring of plasma levels. Since plasma levels of catecholamine are thought to shift suddenly, intermittent sampling techniques such as used now are apt to miss intermittent bursts. The development of enzymatically tipped probes for this purpose would be a great contribution and is conceivable.

CATECHOLAMINE RELEASE IN MAN

Clinical Resting Conditions

True resting conditions for determination of catecholamine excretion are those in which the subject is at minimal physical activity, free from psychic distractions and not ingesting agents stimulating catecholamine release. Such resting conditions are obviously hard to achieve but can be closely approached by an overnight 12 hour urine collection made from 8 p.m. to 8 a.m. During much of this time, the subject will be asleep and during all of this time should be conveniently quiet, lying down in his room.[31] Alcohol should be scrupulously avoided (one predinner cocktail can quadruple the overnight excretion rate of epinephrine and norepinephrine) and smoking should be minimized to a point compatible with psychic ease. Light sedation for sleep is permissible if the patient would otherwise be restless in the strange hospital surroundings without it. If feasible, we wait until the night of the second or third hospital day to make a resting collection. By this time the subject is better acclimatized to the hospital. For most purposes we prefer to make two overnight collections to detect variation in resting excretion.

Specific foodstuffs to be avoided are bananas and avocados since both of these contain catecholamines and VMA. Ingested catecholamines are deaminated and 3-*O*-methylated in the liver and will give falsely high values for VMA. Vanilla flavoring should be avoided since Vanillin is converted to vanillymandillic acid in the liver and elsewhere and gives a false positive value for urinary VMA excretion.

Of medications interfering with catecholamine analysis, the most important is α-methyl-dopa (Aldomet®). This forms a trihydroxyindole ring. False positive urinary and plasma norepinephrine and epinephrine values will result and, although statements to the contrary appear, false positive VMA values can also appear with the use of α-methyl-dopa. Ideally a patient should be free from α-methyl-dopa treatment for at least three weeks before catecholamine studies are done.

Some antibiotics and vitamins have sufficient native fluorescence to be a problem. These appear as fluorogenic substances raising the fluorescent background of sample blanks to unacceptably high levels and can be appreciated immediately.

Urine samples should be collected into a tinted laboratory bottle to which 10 ml, 6 N hydrochloric acid has been added. The pH of the collection should be less than 3.6. These conditions minimize oxidation of the catecholamines for 4 days. This is sufficient time to permit shipping of samples to laboratories for catecholamine analysis.

These few remarks concerning catecholamine sample collection and analysis are made because physicians ordering such determinations on patients under their care cannot do so intelligently unless there is some appreciation of the limitations of the conditions and techniques involved.[30]

Resting Excretion of Epinephrine, Norepinephrine, and Metanephrines

Resting excretion rates, although measured in a 12 hour collection, are for convenience, conventionally calculated and expressed as resting 24 hour excretion of free catecholamines. If impairment of renal function is present or completeness of sample collection is questioned, one can express catecholamine excretion rates as μg of free epinephrine and norepinephrine per milligram of excreted creatinine.

Normal adults excrete, in true resting conditions, norepinephrine 29 $\pm$ 1.2 (1 S.D.) epinephrine and 7.2 $\pm$ 4.2 (1 S.D.) μg per 24 hours. The metanephrines are usually measured as the sum of free and conjugated forms. Twenty-four hour excretion values for these metanephrines are larger than those for free catecholamines being 21 $\pm$ 6 μg free, 223 $\pm$ 68 μg conjugated, 244 μg total for normetanephrine; 30 $\pm$ 6 μg free, 134 $\pm$ 26 μg, conjugated, and 164 μg total, for 24 hours excretion of metanephrine in normal subjects.[30,95]

Stimulated Catecholamine Release from Normal Adrenal Glands and Nerves

Of the many clinical disorders involving the catecholamines and their secretion three are especially pertinent to surgical disease. The three situations are fundamentally different; first, the neuroendocrine response to surgery is a predictable and probably useful adrenergic response; second, sympatholysis in clinical shock represents misguided treatment; third, massive thermal burns represent a fascinating clinical syndrome associated with pathologically high catecholamine secretion rates from normal adrenergic nerves and adrenal chromaffin cells.

There are many other interesting clinical situations associated with augmented catecholamine release which can only be mentioned. Congestive heart failure, muscular exercise, and arteriovenous fistulae all are germane to surgical patients and are associated with catecholamine release.

NEUROENDOCRINE RESPONSE TO SURGERY

The neuroendocrine response to surgery involves the acute hypersecretion of a large complex of the so-called "stress" hormones in response to surgery. Among the hormones often released are epinephrine and norepinephrine and probably dopamine as well. Moore and Franksson have studied this phenomenon and found urinary excretion rates of norepinephrine of approximately 80 μg per day and of epinephrine 20 μg per day, for about 2 days.[36,43] This secretory increase occurred only with large operations or major surgical illness. The increased secretion of other hormones, notably that of hydrocortisone, disappears less rapidly. We suppose that this secretion of catecholamines is purposeful and helpful. At the very least, the increased oxidative energy made available by catecholamine induced glycogenolysis, helps to meet acutely increased energy requirements present after surgery.

Attempts have been made to dissect the variety of stimuli to the endocrine glands inherent in surgery and all that goes with it. Psychic arousal is thought to be the most important stimulus. The studies of Franksson et al.[36] suggest that acute catecholamine release in response to surgery is less frequent than was originally supposed.

Some anesthetic agents, particularly sodium pentothal, can be potent adrenergic stimulants. Others, halothane for example, while irritating to the myocardium are known to decrease levels of plasma catecholamines. Finally, it cannot be overemphasized that the entire constellation of events associated with acute surgical illness of any major kind and its ultimate correction by surgery renders the surgical patient vulnerable to hypoxia at many steps along the way. Hypoventilation during a prolonged operation, pain, and overmedication for pain all may easily produce postoperative hypoxia. A burst of catecholamine release could be expected at any point. Pain stimulates the release of catecholamine perhaps in response to the psychic arousal associated with it. Sudden hemorrhage or plasma volume loss for any reason may be sufficiently great in surgery to stimulate acute release of catecholamines both from the adrenal medulla and peripheral adrenergic nerves.

For all of these reasons it should hardly be surprising that brisk, noticeable adrenal medullary and noradrenergic secretion is often part of the neuroendocrine response in surgery. In certain situations it is of greater concern if this response does not occur. It would be relatively easy to block the major effects of these released catecholamines by any of a variety of sympatholytic regimens. However, there is no reason to do so and it is possible that such categorical treatment would deprive the patient of useful cardiovascular and metabolic adaptations promoting recovery.

SYMPATHOLYSIS IN CLINICAL SHOCK

An excellent example of misplaced categorical therapy is apparent in the attempts to treat clinical shock by adrenolytic drugs. About ten years ago the suggestion was made, and carried out, that clinical shock patterns in man, regardless of their origin, should, if resistant to other forms of treatment, be managed with alpha adrenergic blockade with dibenamine or phenoxybenzamine. The rationale was clear. Tissue perfusion could be improved by relieving peripheral vasoconstriction which was predominantly a result of noradrenergic responses to the shock producing situation. In fact, experimentally and clinically, no hard evidence could be produced to demonstrate fundamental benefit from such treatment. Most shock patients appear to die as easily with high or low peripheral resistance and tissue perfusion. It is significant that no two authors writing about their experience with sympatholytic treatment in shock agreed on the indications for this treatment and a number of surgeons actively advocating alpha adrenergic receptor blockade in shock could not define the precise conditions in which it should be used. Sympatholytic treatment of shock has now virtually disappeared from view and it appears in retrospect that the criteria for initiating such treatment were too diffuse and not specifically drawn. The treatment was more meddlesome than helpful, not critically evaluated and tended to diminish the concentration of the involved physicians on the primary causes of the shock. In addition, it is obvious in retrospect at least, that prior experimental evaluation of the sympatholytic regimens in shock were cursory and not adequately done.

Such skepticism should not prevent imaginative trials of adrenergic blockade in treating uniquely appropriate forms of clinical shock in the future. This is particularly true in conditions in which the indications for treatment are carefully defined. Concomitant alpha adrenergic receptor blockade and norepinephrine infusion in cardiogenic shock is an apt example.

THERMAL BURNS

A fascinating, much studied, and still imperfectly understood pathologic hypersecretion of catecholamines occurs, not infrequently, in patients with large thermal burns. This catecholamine hypersecretion may persist for several months after the burn injury. This hypersecretion is unique in that it represents the relentless excessive secretory response of a fundamentally normal adrenergic nervous system. This catecholamine release can be more dramatic in magnitude and duration than any other we know except in very active pheochromocytoma. There are important effects of this catecholamine release on the burn patients and sometimes specific therapy is required.

In the 1950s it was appreciated at the Karolinska Sjükhuset that patients with large body burns had more than a slight and transient adrenergic burst such as might be expected in the neuroendocrine response to injury. In the burn patients, free excretion rates as high as 550 μg norepinephrine per day and 250 μg epinephrine per day or more were seen. In some cases the phenomenon persisted for as long as 4 to 5 months. Goodall, following his research training in Stockholm, has devoted a major part of his scientific career to the study of this catecholamine hypersecretion in burned patients.

Goodall's earliest publication[40] on burns defined the magnitude and duration of this wild exaggeration of catecholamine release. Many of these patients had a normal blood pressure throughout even though the quantities of catecholamines excreted not infrequently exceeded those of some pheochromocytoma patients, most of whom are flagrantly hypertensive. At the time of Goodall's first report, bioassay techniques for urinary catecholamines were still in widespread use. Bioassay techniques for catecholamines are mainly of historical interest now but gave, at the time, clear definition of the extent of this prolonged catecholamine release. Shortly after Goodall's first report, the Karolinska group published similar findings.[8]

Goodall's next studies were of catecholamine metabolism in affected burn patients. He noted that in a few of the catecholamine hypersecretors, the increased epinephrine and norepinephrine excretion abruptly vanished. These patients tended to be among those who were both more seriously burned and exhibited more complicated, stormy, and prolonged postburn clinical courses. At the time of abrupt cessation of exaggerated catecholamine release the patients deteriorated markedly and died. Goodall demonstrated that exhaustion of catecholamine stores had occurred and felt that administration of a catecholamine precursor (dopamine) might restore the exaggerated catecholamine release.[39] This proved to be the case and the pertinent question became whether or not the burn patients supported in this way in fact survived conditions which would have otherwise been fatal. This is a difficult question to answer and will require years of study to resolve.

Most recently a variety of workers including Goodall have pursued the question of what stimulus there is for this extraordinary adrenergic release. Two factors have been suspected. One is the pain and considerable apprehension that are so prominent in the severely burned. The other is that bacterial toxin absorbed from the burn wound into the systemic circulation could stimulate this release. Bacterial endotoxins are liberated in the burn wound from the huge bacterial populations flourishing there and enter the circulation. It is obvious that intelligently directed preventive and therapeutic measures can be directed against both of these stimuli. It is possible that a hypothalamic adrenergic stimulation is active in these burn patients. This latter view is favored by the sophisticated research group at the Brooke Army Hospital.

Some insights into the consequences of excessive catecholamine secretion on the burn patient have come from entirely separate directions. In 1953 the burn study group at the Massachusetts General Hospital demonstrated persistent hypermetabolism in some severely burned patients. Thyroid function studies were normal in these same patients and it was a puzzle as to why this increased oxygen utilization should occur.[22] Some supposed that there was an abnormal loss of oxygen through the burn wound although this could never be demonstrated; furthermore, the hypermetabolism continued when a well-developed eschar seemed to provide an effective barrier to gas exchange. Sophisticated calorimetric studies by the late Carl Moyer and his associates demonstrated an increased heat energy produced by the burn patient which in fact, required increased oxygen but this did not identify the physiologic stimulus to increased oxygen consumption.[16]

Epinephrine and norepinephrine can have pronounced calorigenic effects and stimulate an increase in oxygen consumption and a statistically significant correlation between elevated catecholamine excretion and hypermetabolism has been found in hypermetabolic burn patients.[58] It seems clear that at least one physiological mechanism driving the burn patient to increased oxygen utilization is increased catecholamine secretion.

Most recently workers at the U.S. Army Burn Research Center at Brooke Army Hospital have noted that in hypermetabolic burn patients, beta adrenergic receptor blockade has converted increased rates of oxygen consumption to normal.[99] Also noted was catecholamine exhaustion and a subsequently serious clinical course following the occurrence of that phenomenon. This is important support of Goodall's original observations.

Some effects of the catecholamines are overtly harmful to burn patients. In burned children, acute hypertensive crises have produced dangerous encephalopathies and death. These hypertensive crises are accompanied by increases in free epinephrine and norepinephrine excretion and the degree of hypertension can be statistically correlated with the magnitude of catecholamine hypersecretion. Vigorous reserpine treatment effectively dissipates this hypertensive crisis and these children now often survive a situation that once was frequently fatal.[45]

For years delayed burn fatalities have been recognized three and four months post injury associated with bizarre syndromes of hepatic insufficiency and myocardial failure. Postmortem examinations of these delayed burn deaths often showed myriads of focal necroses in the liver and myocardium. These same lesions have been produced experimentally by administration of catecholamines and it is logical that catecholamines lie at the heart of the pathophysiologic mechanism involved in these bizarre deaths. A careful retrospective study of fatal burns could provide valuable insight into whether or not excessive catecholamine release is an important feature of this problem.

AUTONOMOUS HYPERSECRETION OF CATECHOLAMINES IN MAN: PHEOCHROMOCYTOMA

Pathophysiology

Up to this point we have considered catecholamine release as a phenomenon occurring from catecholamine storage sites in chromaffin cells of the innervated adrenal medulla and from functioning peripheral postganglionic adrenergic nerves. We now turn to a distinctly different phenomenon, that of production and release of dopamine, norepinephrine and epinephrine from benign and malignant tumors of chromaffin cells. The chromaffin cells of these tumors are not innervated and the factors governing catecholamine release from them are independent of the nervous system's reflex control. This autonomous release of catecholamines is not well understood, but there are a few helpful insights.

The chromaffin cells of pheochromocytomas synthesize norepinephrine from tyrosine and contain the requisite enzymes for this. About one-third of the pheochromocytomas can synthesize epinephrine as well; this final step in the synthesis probably depends on the availability of cortisol to the tumor cells.

The primary release of catecholamines from these tumors eludes precise understanding. A few pheochromocytomas excrete free dopamine in the urine and rarely dopa (dihydroxyphenylalanine) can be identified.[91] Dopa excretion has been considered to be an indication of malignancy in pheochromocytoma but there are many exceptions and the phenomenon of dopa excretion itself is too rare to be of practical help in identifying all malignant chromaffin cell tumors.

Once catecholamines are released from pheochromocytomas, they are subject to the same mechanisms for metabolic and physiologic termination that inactivate physiologically released catecholamines. This includes uptake into neuronal storage pools. The absolute quantity of circulating catecholamine is greatly increased in pheochromocytoma with arterial plasma content of norepinephrine and epinephrine commonly ten times normal values. Whether or not tissue levels of catecholamines in pheochromocytoma are raised in response to chronically increased plasma levels of epinephrine and norepinephrine is an interesting question. We have measured hepatic norepinephrine and epinephrine content in five pheochromocytoma patients and found, in four, significant elevations of the same catecholamines being excessively excreted in the urine.

Given the likelihood that catecholamine tissue levels are increased in pheochromocytoma[52] one can logically ask whether such increased tissue stores respond to conventional reflex stimuli by releasing increased quantities of dopamine, norepinephrine, and epinephrine. A safe and convenient reflex stimulus for this purpose is the tilt test. In this test, urinary catecholamine excretion is determined for a 3-hour period with the subject lying flat. The patient supported by a foot board is then tilted to a plus 75° head up position, encouraged to take fluids and voids a second time after another 3 hours have passed. Normal subjects studied in this way increase their urinary norepinephrine and epinephrine excretion in the erect position.[31] This is considered to be a reflex mediated by volume receptors in the great veins and right atrium stimulated by the contraction of these vessels associated with the postural shifts of the central blood volume. This is probably the same afferent stimulus as that involved in the catecholamine response to acute hemorrhage.

Almost all pheochromocytoma patients do respond to the tilt test with an exaggerated release of free norepinephrine or epinephrine into the urine.[50] Exaggerated release of dopamine occurred as well in the two pheochromocytomas in whom it was studied. This heightened response usually disappears within a week after pheochromocytoma removal.

Scrupulously minded pharmacologists have been reluctant to ascribe this phenomenon of exaggerated catecholamine release in pheochromocytoma to heightened reflex response from increased catecholamine stores. This would, in their view, violate the quantal concept of catecholamine release originally set forward by Sir Lindor Brown and others.[12] In essence this concept, and there is good physiologic support for it with normal catecholamine stores, maintains that for each adrenergic nerve impulse reaching catecholamine storage sites, there is a finite number of molecules of catecholamine released into the circulation. Why then, in the pharmacologist's view, does heightened reflex release occur in pheochromocytoma? They feel that postural changes of the tilt test place traction on the tumor and this stimulates catecholamine release directly from the tumor. There are reasons to doubt that this explanation is uniformly suitable, but little would be gained by developing the question further with the information presently at hand. The entire question of reflex release from chronically oversaturated stores of catecholamines remains one of great theoretical and practical interest and requires more investigation.

There can be great variation in catecholamine excretion rates from one day to the next in a given pheochromocytoma patient. No adequate explanation has been made for this but the variation can be correlated with concomitant changes in the patient's clinical course. At the time pheochromocytoma patients are the most ill their catecholamine excretion rates tend to be high.[51]

In pheochromocytoma, not a small number of patients have elevated levels of plasma renin activity. Originally the plasma renin elevation was found in pheochromocytoma patients whose tumor was compressing the renal artery.[96] More recently elevated renin has been demonstrated in other pheochromocytomas that are not compressing the renal artery. This phenomenon is most often seen with norepinephrine secreting lesions and it is felt that the norepinephrine produces a great enough vasoconstriction of the renal circulation to produce a Goldblatt Phenomenon from constricted small intrarenal resistance vessels.[75,97] Furthermore, many of the pheochromocytoma patients with elevated plasma renin values also have contracted plasma volume; this situation is known to stimulate renin release. In several of our patients with elevated plasma renin values, we have measured plasma renin after preoperative blockade with phenoxybenzamine. At the time of measurement, the plasma volume has returned to normal as judged by resolution of the hematocrit to normal values. At this time, there has been a substantial decrease in the plasma renin concentration toward but not all the way to normal. Our current feeling is that there is frequently an element of adrenergic stimulation and plasma volume contraction combining to cause the elevation in plasma renin activity seen in pheochromocytoma patients.

In one of our patients, a child with malignant hypertension, there were massive increases in both norepinephrine excretion and plasma renin activity. Nine months after tumor removal there was again a large increase in norepinephrine excretion and at that time both plasma renin and blood pressure were normal.[53] This suggests that in this patient the increased blood pressure was related more closely to the plasma renin levels than to increases in catecholamine excretion.

Released catecholamines are not metabolized with the same efficiency in pheochromocytoma as in normal man.[52] In man a normal ratio of 0.067, 20 μg, norepinephrine per 300 μg normetanephrine was increased to 0.400, 4,200 μg norepinephrine per 10,500 μg, normetanephrine in one of our more actively secreting pheochromocytoma patients. The same phenomenon can be demonstrated in patients with tumors secreting predominantly epinephrine, a normal 0.031 ratio, 5 μg, epinephrine per 160 μg, metanephrine, being increased to 0.333, 1,000 μg, epinephrine per 3,000 μg, metanephrine per 24 hours. A less active lesion secreting predominantly epinephrine demonstrated a normal ratio 0.027, 16.3, epinephrine μg per 612 metanephrine. In this latter case the tumor was less active than many others and the capacity of the *O*-methyl-transferase system was not exceeded.

In two patients with norepinephrine secreting tumors responding to the tilt test with large increases in norepinephrine excretion there was no simultaneous rise in the excretion rate of normetanephrine during the same tilt test. This is good evidence in man that if metanephrines are present in intraneuronal storage sites they are not released from such storage sites by reflex activity. We have seen heightened release of alpha-methyl-norepinephrine, a false transmitter, in response to the tilt test in a patient who had been receiving chronic alpha-methyl-dopa treatment.[50]

Diagnosis

BIOCHEMICAL TESTS FOR PHEOCHROMOCYTOMA

The presence of pheochromocytoma is usually suspected in any patient with episodic hypertension. There are, however, patients with sustained hypertension who harbor the tumor and rarely asymptomatic patients who have had pheochromocytomas discovered. Furthermore, in recent years many patients suspected of having a pheochromocytoma have been referred with a classical history of episodic hypertensive attacks, sweating, apprehension, and palpitations. Often one or two noncritical diagnostic tests have been positive and the patient is referred for surgery with the diagnosis of pheochromocytoma already "established" by uncritical evidence. Most often these patients turn out not to have a pheochromocytoma.

Only an estimated 0.1 percent of hypertensives have a pheochromocytoma and a larger proportion of the hypertensive population have episodic blood pressure shifts. Ideally the possibility of pheochromocytoma should be excluded in every person with high blood pressure since it is one of the curable forms of hypertension and there are definite

Table 3-1
Free Catecholamine and Metanephrine Excretion in Hypertensive Suspects (normal) and Patients with Demonstrated Pheochromocytoma

	Normal (n = 100)		Pheochromocytoma (n = 63)
Norepinephrine	28.9[a] ± 29.0[b]	(P < 0.001)	1250 ± 2456
Epinephrine	7.6 ± 7.4	(P < 0.001)	238 ± 408
	Normal (n = 37)		Pheochromocytoma (n = 29)
Normetanephrine	44.2 ± 38.9	(P < 0.001)	1127 ± 842
Metanephrine	32.9 ± 16.4	(P < 0.001)	1305 ± 1708

[a] All urinary values in micrograms per 24 hours.
[b] ±1 Standard deviation.
By permission from, Freier and Harrison, ref. 37.

risks associated with leaving pheochromocytomas unattended. It is estimated that in the United States each year between 600 to 800 cases of pheochromocytoma occur.

For all of these reasons, it is imperative that rigorous diagnostic criteria be available to establish as definitely as possible the presence of pheochromocytoma. Currently such criteria are best satisfied by measuring the free urinary excretion of norepinephrine, epinephrine, normetanephrine, and metanephrine. It is important that the subjects be studied in resting conditions. We customarily make two overnight 12 hour urine collections.

This approach to diagnosis has been accurate in 67 urine samples of 28 pheochromocytoma patients whose lesions have ultimately been demonstrated at operation and confirmed microscopically.[37] Thirty-seven of these urines were analyzed for the metanephrines as well. The results are summarized in Table 3-1. There have been, and others have had this experience as well, occasional patients, less than 10 percent, with normal epinephrine and norepinephrine excretion rates, who nevertheless have persistent elevation of either normetanephrine or metanephrine depending upon the secretory profile of the tumor. These patients ultimately prove to have pheochromocytomas and we can infer that their *O*-methyl-transferase enzyme activity is equal to the increased demands made on it by the large quantities of catecholamines released from the tumor.[11]

We have had no instance of normal metanephrine and/or normetanephrine excretion in a pheochromocytoma patient. Others have had this experience as well; rare borderline cases are now beginning to appear, especially in the study of congenital asymptomatic pheochromocytoma suspects such as patients with Sipple's syndrome. There is no reason to suppose that borderline diagnostic situations will not task and bedevil our insight into this situation more and more as we continue to sharpen our diagnostic precision and awareness for pheochromocytoma. We turned down two patients for surgery because of repeated normal excretion of norepinephrine, epinephrine, normetanephrine, and metanephrine. The patients were ultimately explored by other surgeons. In one case, free total catecholamines (norepinephrine + epinephrine) showed borderline elevations coinciding with intense agitation and associated physical exercise. No pheochromocytomas were found in either of these two patients. We are aware of two other similar situations in which negative explorations have been made.

Currently attempts are being made in some clinics to stimulate, usually with histamine or glucagon, diagnostic rises in plasma norepinephrine and epinephrine in borderline cases. Far too little data on normal subjects' plasma catecholamine response to these stimuli is available to know how useful this will be in the diagnosis of borderline pheochromocytomas with equivocal urinary findings.

False positive elevations in norepinephrine, epinephrine, normetanephrine, and metanephrine excretion have been rare and can generally be resolved by repeated study on separate hospitalizations, sometimes months apart and insistence on true resting conditions as defined before.

In many laboratory groups around the world, a large effort has been made to use the determination of urinary vanillylmandelic acid (VMA) excretion as a diagnostic test in pheochromocytoma. In addition, this has been suggested as a screening device to survey large hypertensive populations for the presence of occult pheochromocytoma. The logic of using VMA excretion for this purpose is inescapable; VMA is the end metabolic product of norepinephrine and epinephrine metabolism and is excreted free in the urine in at least 100 times the quantity of norepinephrine and epinephrine.

However, some serious problems have arisen with VMA determination in pheochromocytoma. Many of these difficulties relate to the colorimetric reaction for measuring VMA which is a poor analytical test. The newer VMA techniques which partially overcome this are too laborious for the routine and widespread laboratory use necessary in an ideal screening test.

Half of our pheochromocytoma patients have had a normal VMA excretion demonstrated at some time during their preoperation evaluation and other laboratories have had the same experience.[51,89] This point is of more than casual interest. The death of a hypertensive mother at term and of her baby were recently reported both of which can be directly attributed to false negative VMA values during a "hypertension of pregnancy." Anesthesia was induced for a caesarean section because of fetal distress. The anesthesia course was stormy with wide fluctuations in blood pressure and both baby and mother died during the operation. At autopsy of the mother a right adrenal pheochromocytoma was found.[21] Clinically the diagnosis of pheochromocytoma was considered early in the course of pregnancy and excluded twice on the basis of normal VMA excretion rates. There is no reason to doubt that the diagnosis could have been made successfully with the determination of catecholamine and metanephrine excretions. Had this been done adequate preoperative measures, particularly partial adrenergic receptor blockade, could have minimized the risk to the mother and her baby.

PHARMACOLOGIC TESTS FOR PHEOCHROMOCYTOMA

The literature on pheochromocytoma of the past 30 years is filled with a variety of diagnostic tests which depend on pharmacologic stimulation of exaggerated blood pressure increase in pheochromocytoma or on a blood pressure fall following intravenous sympatholytic drugs.

Agents stimulating catecholamine release used in the past include histamine, tryamine, glucagon, and cold. If a pheochromocytoma is present the blood pressure rise will be more than that in subjects without pheochromocytoma. There are two reasons to predict that this diagnostic approach might be troublesome. First of all, the success of the stimulating tests in general depends upon uniformly increased reactivity, in terms of catecholamine release, of pheochromocytoma patients to a given drug. Secondly, assuming that a certain diagnostically increased quantity of catecholamine is released, a standard reactivity of all pheochromocytoma patients to released catecholamines must be present. This latter phenomenon is known not to be true as evidenced in the small percentage of pheochromocytoma patients known to have normal blood pressure coincidentally with large increases in urinary catecholamine excretion.

For these reasons it is hardly surprising that there is a conspicuous false negative rate, about 30 percent, with all stimulating tests in pheochromocytoma. The converse is true also, namely that 10 to 15 percent of hypertensive patients under investigation for pheochromocytoma exhibit diagnostically great blood pressure responses to whatever drug is being used but in fact turn out not to have any other evidence for pheochromocytoma. Some of these patients have been explored and no tumor has been found.

A second objection to pharmacologic stimulation for diagnosis is that, in some pheochromocytoma patients, excessive catecholamine release occurs and deaths have resulted from acute hypertensive reactions. Availability of intravenous adrenergic blocking agents, notably phentolamine, will minimize this risk but such a pharmacologic tug of war is, in our opinion, inherently too risky to be appropriate. It would be hard to support this degree of manipulation for a good diagnostic test in pheochromocytoma and there is no support for maneuvers of this magnitude for highly inaccurate diagnostic tests. In a recent series of seven patients with pheochromocytoma, the glucagon test was positive in all seven, but the test had to be interrupted with intravenous phentolamine in two.[93] Others, it must be noted, have had less success with the glucagon test and have encountered the same risk of provoking an acute hypertensive crisis.

A blocking test with intravenous phentolamine (Regitine®) has, and continues to enjoy widespread use in pheochromocytoma. If the blood pressure falls significantly a diagnosis of pheochromocytoma is made. The error rate of this test is also unacceptably high, about 30 percent false positive and almost as many false negative reactions in patients who ultimately prove to have pheochromocytomas. Even more important are a number of deaths from profound, irreversible hypotension which have occurred in pheochromocytoma patients who over respond to the dose of phentolamine used. The hypotension is refractory to all measures including norepinephrine infusion. Use of smaller doses of Regitine makes the test more ambiguous and increases its unacceptability for that reason.

SCREENING TESTS FOR PHEOCHROMOCYTOMA

Acute fatal hypertensive crisis, dangerous or fatal hypertensive crisis excited during anesthesia for unrelated diseases, and fatal hypotension following massive spontaneous hemorrhage into a pheochromocytoma all still occur in modern medical practice in patients with occult pheochromocytoma. These are patients in whom the diagnosis of pheochromocytoma has not been suspected. It would be to the point to screen, not just the entire hypertensive population but all patients for the possibility of occult pheochromocytoma.

At present there is no adequate screening test for pheochromocytoma. If urinary collections are made it is essential that they be obtained under true resting conditions and this is not compatible with mass screening. Furthermore, determination of urinary catecholamines, metanephrines and VMA is too laborious for widespread screening unless a large investment in effort and expense is made.

In most hospitals, including our own, it has not yet been possible to adequately study most of the hypertensive population of out-patients coming to the hospital, let alone the entire out-patient population. It is estimated that one or two in each thousand hypertensive patients will have a pheochromocytoma. During an eight year period in which we have operated on 28 patients, three patients with unsuspected and unrecognized pheochromocytoma have succumbed from acute hypertensive attacks in our hospital. Their lesions have been demonstrated at autopsy. Therefore, we know that for every 10 patients we have treated there is at least one pheochromocytoma escaping detection. We probably see more patients on referral than the usual hospital which treats hypertensive patients so there is reason to suspect that the ratio of treated to untreated pheochromocytomas is even greater in the population at large. Since 600 to 800 new cases of pheochromocytoma are treated in the United States each year, we think that in this country at least 80 people die yearly from undetected pheochromocytoma. This reasoning is the crux of the argument for widespread pheochromocytoma screening. As will be discussed, the risk inherent in surgery for pheochromocytoma is between 5 to 10 percent for all pheochromocytomas and is now less than 5 percent for primary elective pheochromocytoma excision. It is safer, by far, to have the diagnosis made and the lesions removed. This, in our mind, makes application of a true screening procedure for pheochromocytoma an urgent matter.

Our own interest in this aspect of pheochromocytoma has centered on developing a radioimmunoassay for plasma normetanephrine and metanephrine. In theory the determination of plasma metanephrines should be well suited for pheochromocytoma screening. Use of plasma norepinephrine and epinephrine for pheochromocytoma screening is conceivable but it seems likely to us that this will produce false positive elevations in situations underlying random sample collection of blood plasma. Factors such as physical activity, the erect posture all occur at times of blood collection as does the apprehension of being stuck with a needle. All of these might be predicted to contribute to other than a true resting state and to confuse the significance of borderline elevations of circulating catecholamines. Plasma metanephrines are less apt to reflect these limitations and it would be desirable to have critical evaluation of this point on a large normal population.

Blood samples are far more conveniently collected than urine and it is likely that diagnostic elevations of metanephrines would occur in the plasma of pheochromocytoma patients. In fact, the technical complexity of a radioimmunoassay for plasma metanephrines is formidable and we have not yet mastered it. Other laboratory groups have sought to develop a radioimmunoassay for plasma norepinephrine and epinephrine. This too is proving to be a difficult technical problem but there is no reason to doubt that these techniques will eventually be established. Gas chromatography can be used for determining these compounds but is far too time consuming and elaborate a procedure for large scale screening.[20] As much can be said for the double isotope method for the determination of plasma catecholamines.[25]

Preoperative Evaluation and Care in Pheochromocytoma

BACKGROUND

Once the diagnosis of pheochromocytoma is established the goal of the physician is, obviously, to create optimum conditions for the ultimate safe removal of the tumor. In the early days of surgery for this disease, that is until 20 years ago, the situation of pheochromocytoma removal was often hazardous because massive release of catecholamines occurred during anesthesia and surgery and there were wide fluctuations in blood pressure. Myocardial irritability with refractory dysrhythmias of the heart, especially ventricular fibrillation, were commonly seen and difficult to reverse. If these pitfalls could be successfully avoided there were still apt to be great difficulties at the time of tumor removal because manipulation of the tumor could cause a marked release of catecholamines. Finally, after the venous drainage of the tumor was ligated a circulation chronically acclimatized and well adapted to hugely excessive quantities of catecholamines reaching its adrenergic vascular receptors was suddenly deprived of this excessive quantity of catecholamines. Sudden, profound hypotension immediately after excision of the tumor or ligation of its major veins was seen frequently. Generally this hypotension responded to aggressive blood volume replacement of surprising proportions, sometimes 4 to 5,000 ml of blood or plasma expander or electrolyte solution being required. We now recognize that these patients developed at the time of tumor excision, a sudden passive dilatation of their adrenergically stimulated capacitance vessels such as the spleen and great veins, because they were suddenly deprived of the excessive norepinephrine or epinephrine reaching these vascular receptors. Most often such reactions responded to the volume replacement mentioned but if not norepinephrine infusion was required, generally for 24 to 36 hours.

It is hardly surprising that in this old era of treatment, pheochromocytoma excision was looked upon as a highly dangerous undertaking associated with an operative mortality described by some surgical groups as being 30 to 40 percent. The advent of selective preoperative partial alpha and beta adrenergic receptor blockade in pheochromocytoma has changed this picture markedly.

PREOPERATIVE ALPHA AND BETA ADRENERGIC RECEPTOR BLOCKADE IN PHEOCHROMOCYTOMA

Operative mortality and stormy early postoperative courses are now the exception rather than the rule in the surgical treatment of pheochromocytoma.[66,80,84] An important reason for this is the development of preoperative alpha and beta adrenergic receptor blockade. This treatment is carried out for days and often for weeks before surgery and if used intelligently will result in smooth, dependable cardiovascular dynamics during the period of anesthesia induction, during surgical removal of the pheochromocytoma and in the early postoperative period.

The intelligent use of both alpha and beta receptor blockade in pheochromocytoma requires some awareness of the theory of adrenergic receptors and appreciation of the major effects of norepinephrine and epinephrine on these receptors.

The concept of chemical transmission of an electrical impulse from nerve to effector cell was originally described by T. R. Elliott in 1904. Dale in 1933 and Ahlquist in 1948 further clarified the role of the adrenergic nervous system. Their observations explained the common features of epinephrine responsiveness exhibited by a variety of organs. The aptness of their observations and the concepts derived from them was supported by the discovery of endogenous norepinephrine by U. S. von Eueler and Holtz simultaneously in the late 1940s.

The degree of vasodilatation or vasoconstriction produced by epinephrine depends upon the concentration and number of beta receptor sites available. Epinephrine more readily activates beta receptors at low concentrations but can produce intense activation of alpha receptors at high concentrations. Norepinephrine on the other hand activates beta receptors of most blood vessels much less intensely than does epinephrine. The activation of alpha receptors by norepinephrine predominates in all vessels except the coronary arteries. The actions of endogenous adrenergic amines upon the heart are mediated in all instances by beta receptor activation with the exception of the coronary vessels which can be constricted slightly by alpha receptor activity. It is noteworthy that pressor actions of adrenergic amines predispose to cardiac arrhythmias. Therefore, a cardiac arrhythmia may derive either from an alpha adrenergic pressor receptor or from direct myocardial beta adrenergic receptor stimulation resulting from excessive circulating catecholamines.[57]

In the conditions of chronic catecholamine excess, a unique feature of pheochromocytoma, certain precautions in the use of alpha and beta receptor blockade need to be kept in mind. Overdoses of propanolol, the most commonly used beta receptor blocking agent, have been fatal to two pheochromocytoma patients of which we are aware. One patient died preoperatively and one succumbed from a cardiac standstill during the induction of anesthesia. All attempts at resuscitation were ineffective. Unfortunately neither of these cases have been reported but in both the doses of propanolol used were in ranges frequently employed for other clinical conditions, i.e., angina pectoris, or resistant tachycardias of hyperthyroidism, etc. The doses were, obviously, excessive for pheochromocytoma. To make the point another way, in pheochromocytoma beta adrenergic receptors are unusually sensitive to blockade by propanolol. Doses of propanolol which are suboptimal for other conditions, e.g., 15 mg four times a day, achieve the maximum acceptable blockade in pheochromocytoma as judged by resolution of sinus tachycardia to rates of 90 beats per minute.

Some workers have used alpha receptor blockade with pheoxybenzamine as a preoperative routine in all pheochromocytoma patients regardless of their preoperative cardiovascular status, volemic state and regardless of what catecholamines are being secreted in excess by the tumor. We mistrust this categorical approach and have developed definite criteria for the use of these potentially dangerous pharmacologic agents as preoperative measures in pheochromocytoma. These criteria are shown in Table 3-2. Using this selective approach we have found

Table 3-2
Clinical Indications for Adrenergic Receptor Blockade in Pheochromocytoma

Indications for Preoperative Alpha Adrenergic Receptor Blockade in Pheochromocytoma
Blood pressure >200/130
Frequent, severe uncontrolled hypertensive attacks
Pronounced decrease in plasma volume, i.e., hematocrit >50 vol percent
Use of beta adrenergic receptor blockade
Indications for Preoperative Beta Adrenergic Receptor Blockade in Pheochromocytoma
Pulse rate >130 per minute
Any history of cardiac arrhythmia
Demonstration of persistent ventricular extra systoles
Tumors secreting predominantly, >75 percent, epinephrine

(By permission from, Harrison et al., ref. 57.)

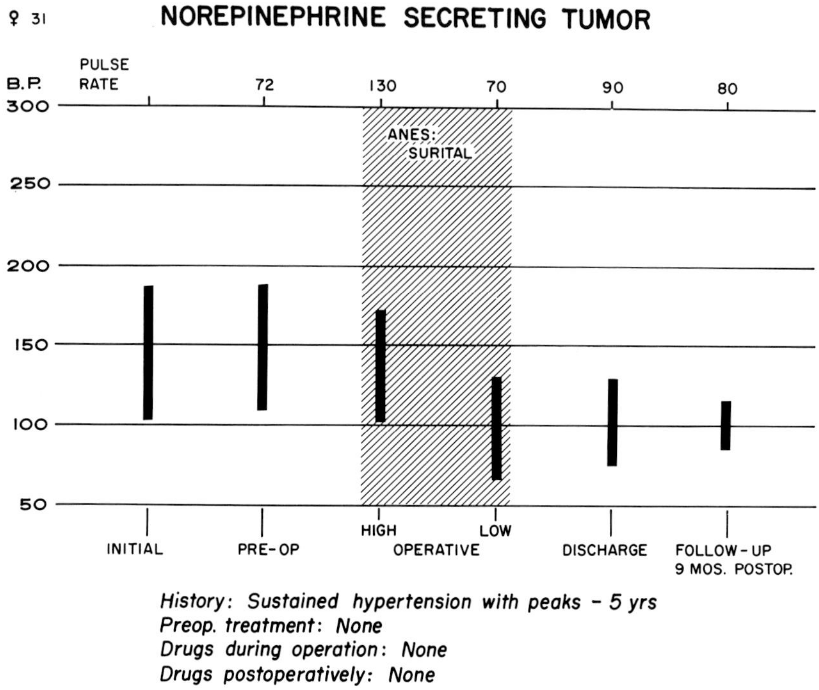

Fig. 3-3. Clinical features of the course of a patient with a norepinephrine secreting pheochromocytoma who did not meet our criteria for preoperative adrenergic receptor blockade. (Reprinted by permission from Harrison et al., ref. 51)

it necessary to block preoperatively only one-half to two-thirds of pheochromocytoma patients and in those who have not been blocked, there has been no reason to wish, retrospectively, that we had done so. In Figure 3-3 the important cardiovascular features of a pheochromocytoma patient's course without blockade are shown. This was a patient with a predominantly norepinephrine secreting tumor, sustained hypertension, and no clinical suggestion of a contracted blood volume. To have added preoperative adrenergic receptor blockade to this situation was not necessary, potentially harmful, and would have contributed nothing further to an already smooth course. Approximately half of our patients with predominantly norepinephrine secreting tumors have not required blockade.[51]

Unquestionably the hypotension seen immediately after tumor excision is prevented in pheochromocytoma patients with contracted blood volumes if preoperative alpha adrenergic blockade has been used. The preoperative alpha receptor stimulated contraction of capacitance vessels is definite when it occurs. However it does not occur as often as most people have supposed and in fact, when blood volume measurements are made in pheochromocytoma only 15 to 25 percent of the patients are found to have diminished plasma volume.[89] For the other 75 percent of pheochromocytoma patients routine alpha adrenergic receptor blockade is potentially meddlesome unless unstable blood pressures or cardiac arrhythmias are present.

Patients under our care whose tumors secrete a mixture of norepinephrine and epinephrine have, with one exception, not required preoperative blockade by our criteria. We believe that there is a crudely balanced overstimulation both of alpha and beta cardiovascular adrenergic receptors in this situation. This may help maintain a stable circulation in which active vasoconstriction, alpha receptor mediated, and active vasodilatation, beta receptor mediated, occur simultaneously.

We have had several occasions to be grateful for the protection afforded by preoperative partial beta receptor blockade. Preoperative arrhythmias such as ventricular extrasystoles, ventricular tachycardias, and runs of ventricular tachycardia are all well known as part of the clinical picture particularly in patients with predominantly epinephrine secreting pheochromocytomas. Not infrequently these arrhythmias may be pressure induced and will respond to preoperative alpha adrenergic receptor blockade. If that is true there is little reason to add beta adrenergic blockade in patients with norepinephrine secreting tumors or tumors that secrete a mixture of norepinephrine and epinephrine.

Early in our experience we had one occasion to regret not using preoperative beta adrenergic receptor blockade. This was in a patient who had a predominantly epinephrine secreting lesion and the tumor, diffusely recurrent, could not be removed. She died 4 hours postoperatively from a combination of acute congestive failure and refractory hypotension. Interestingly enough she had tolerated three previous abdominal explorations for pheochromocytoma perfectly well without adrenergic receptor blockade. The intense beta adrenergic receptor stimulation associated with large excesses of epinephrine is too great a threat to the strength and stability of myocardial contraction and too apt to override peripheral alpha receptor mediated vasoconstriction to ignore. Hence, we now use partial preoperative beta receptor blockade in all patients with predominantly epinephrine secreting tumors. Furthermore, we feel that since the heart with partial beta receptor blockade will respond imperfectly to the increased load imposed by heightened vascular resistance concomitant alpha adrenergic blockade should always be used in conjunction with the beta receptor blockade. A recent patient on

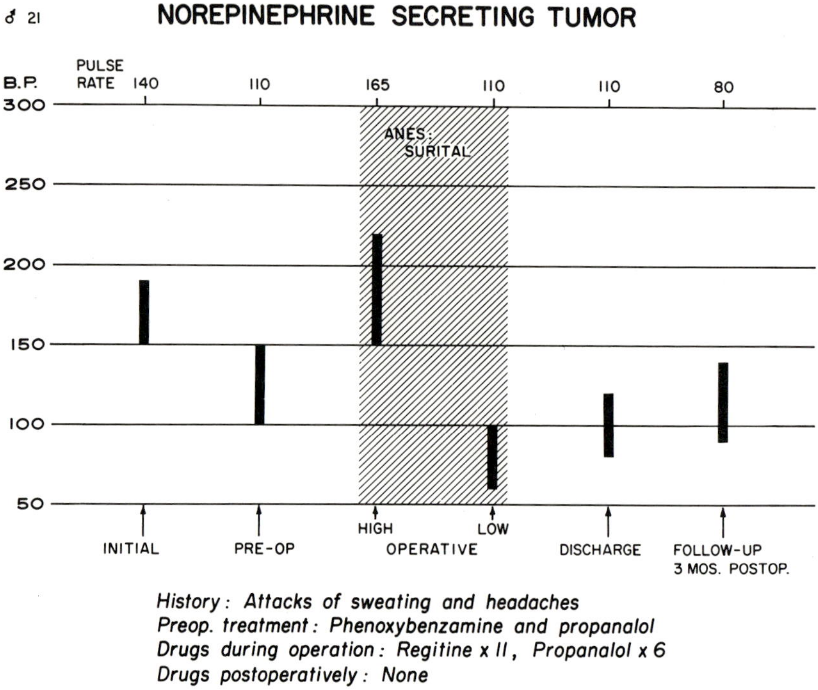

Fig. 3-4. The effects of incomplete blockade are apparent. (Reprinted by permission from Harrison et al., ref. 51.)

whom we were consulted was acutely ill from a predominantly epinephrine secreting lesion. He had been treated with acute intravenous beta receptor blockade only. The pulse rate slowed, the blood pressure became unobtainable and the patient lost consciousness probably from an associated acute decrease in cardiac output.

One important emphasis should be made concerning preoperative adrenergic receptor blockade in pheochromocytoma. This is that large variations occur from one patient to the next in the amount of alpha or beta receptor blocking agent required. Therefore, it is necessary to begin treatment with doses of recognized safety, e.g., no more than 1 mg per kg body weight per day phenoxybenzamine by mouth and 45 mg propanolol per day given in three or four divided doses. These can be increased generally at 4 day intervals until satisfactory resolution of blood pressure and tachycardia have been achieved. An example of the stormy course resulting from incomplete adrenergic receptor blockade is shown in Figure 3-4.

A final point pertaining to preoperative blockade is that uncommonly pheochromocytoma patients are seen with a fulminating clinical picture of sudden exaggeration of the intensity and frequency of their attacks and coincident exaggeration of their hypertension. Attempts to achieve effective partial adrenergic receptor blockade in these patients may be unsuccessful, probably because of the large acute secretory bursts of catecholamines from the tumor. This situation has been termed "acute pheochromocytoma" and can be successfully managed by surgery when it is clear that other measures are not going to be successful.[24] Acute pheochromocytoma has an appreciable risk associated with it.

GENERAL MEASURES IN PREOPERATIVE CARE OF PHEOCHROMOCYTOMA

A large part of the successful care of pheochromocytoma falls into the category of well-informed, vigorous, up-to-date care of the critically ill. This is so much part of the fabric of contemporary medical education and graduate training that there is little need or justification for developing it here. Adequate oxygen delivered to tissues deprived of it in the critically ill and all the clinical awareness required for this are part of the armamentarium of every well educated physician.

However, two features of pheochromocytoma are of special interest and are mentioned for that reason. One feature concerns fluid balance. A few patients with the acute pheochromocytoma syndrome mentioned previously have extremely restricted vascular capacitance. An adult patient under our care with a mixed norepinephrine and epinephrine secreting tumor was acutely ill with a fever of 103°, marked ileus and leukocytosis. Hemoconcentration was evident with a hematocrit of 57 volumes percent. Attempts to expand the plasma volume with electrolyte solutions and/or blood plasma invariably resulted in elevation of central venous pressure and mild pulmonary edema. Only 800 ml of intravenous fluid could be tolerated per day without difficulty. If less than that quantity was given, serious hypotension developed and with appreciably more fluid, recurrent pulmonary edema became a problem.

Digitalis treatment was instituted and the patient's pheochromocytoma removed. Postoperatively, fluid retention with peripheral edema was a problem until a moderate hypoalbuminemia was corrected. After that the patient accepted intravenous and oral fluids without difficulty and continued to do so for the remainder of her course. Digitalis was discontinued postoperatively without any difficulty. The patient had a prolonged course characterized by steady improvement and is well 7 years following removal of her pheochromocytoma.

The other feature of preoperative care of special interest in pheochromocytoma illustrated by this patient concerns the use of digitalis and related drugs in this disease. Epinephrine in particular makes the myocardium and especially the cardiac conduction system sensitive to arrhythmias of all varieties. Digitalis-like drugs can be irritating to the myocardium. Hence, great care must be taken when adding digitalis to the preoperative regimen in pheochromocytoma. Our approach has been never to withhold digitalis or related drugs in pheochromocytoma if there is clearcut evidence of congestive failure, refractory to other measures. We have avoided using rapid digitalization with intravenously administered digitoxin even in the face of failure but rather have proceeded cautiously with orally given drugs over three or four days until full digitalization has been achieved. We have had no problems with this approach and have always been able to maintain full digitalization as long as it was considered necessary.

PREOPERATIVE LOCALIZATION OF PHEOCHROMOCYTOMA

Once the diagnosis of pheochromocytoma is established it is worthwhile preoperatively to have as accurate an idea as possible of the location, number, and size of the tumor(s). Some workers have proceeded to abdominal exploration once the diagnosis has been made but in our view if one knows where the major tumors are located surgical excision can be directed at the known lesion and a deliberate exploration for others can be made under conditions safer than those existing when the tumor is in place.

A variety of localization procedures have been developed over the years and require brief comment. Rarely (2 of 28 cases) can a pheochromocytoma be palpated on physical examination. One of these was a recurrent lesion near the urinary bladder and easily palpable as a left adnexal mass on pelvic examination. Palpation of the tumor did not elicit a hypertensive response. The other palpable mass was a large pheochromocytoma of the right adrenal. Whenever this mass was palpated and whenever the patient lay on his abdomen, a marked hypertensive attack followed.

Plain abdominal x-rays rarely reveal the definite silhouette of pheochromocytoma. The lesion must be large and relatively free from superimposition of other shadows.

Retroperitoneal Gas Insufflation. Presacral gas insufflation often brings the contour of the adrenal glands into sharp relief and may reveal lesions 3 to 4 cm in diameter if they are favorably oriented to the plane of the x-ray. The resolution of this technique can be improved further if laminographic films are made.

Presacral gas insufflation has been virtually abandoned in the United States because of early fatalities from its use. These resulted from occasional entry of the air used into retroperitoneal veins and into the circulation in general and rarely a full blown picture of fatal air embolism developed. The use of gases soluble in blood, carbon dioxide in particular, for this examination has made the technique perfectly safe once again and although it has never regained popularity in the United States it is widely employed, safely and advantageously in Europe, particularly in the major French clinics.

Excretory Urography and Nephrotomography. Intravenous pyelography with visualization of the kidneys, collecting systems, renal pelvices, and ureters has, and continues to enjoy, widespread use in pheochromocytoma workups. Even when combined with nephrotomography, the return from this procedure is disappointingly low. Occasionally large lesions can be seen in or near the adrenal and less often subtle indentation of the ureter or renal pelvices have tipped us off to ectopically located pheochromocytomas. Most frequently nothing dependable is seen.

Most of our patients still have intravenous pyelography performed and perhaps a case can be made for it as a routine evaluation of renal function in patients with long standing hypertension. Seldom does pyelography give definitive information on localization of pheochromocytoma.

Arteriography. Selective and subselective arteriography occasionally may demonstrate convincingly the arterial supply and tumor "stains" associated with lesions greater than 3 cm in diameter. Frequently however, ectopic lesions are smaller than this and there are many instances in which the arteriographic findings are highly suggestive but nevertheless, sufficiently ambiguous so that substantiation by a more definitive localizing technique becomes necessary. Radiographic subtraction techniques may be of some help in this particular regard, Figure 3-5, and the use of vasoactive agents such as angiotensin II may increase the visualization of the tumor.[81,82]

A word of caution must be made concerning the use of arteriography. Angiographic dye can stimulate the release of catecholamines from chromaffin cells and violent hypertensive reactions have occurred. Deaths have resulted from arteriography in pheochromocytoma patients. We use arteriography not infrequently and insist that a functioning indwelling venous catheter be in place during the procedure and that phentolamine be immediately available for use if necessary. In approximately

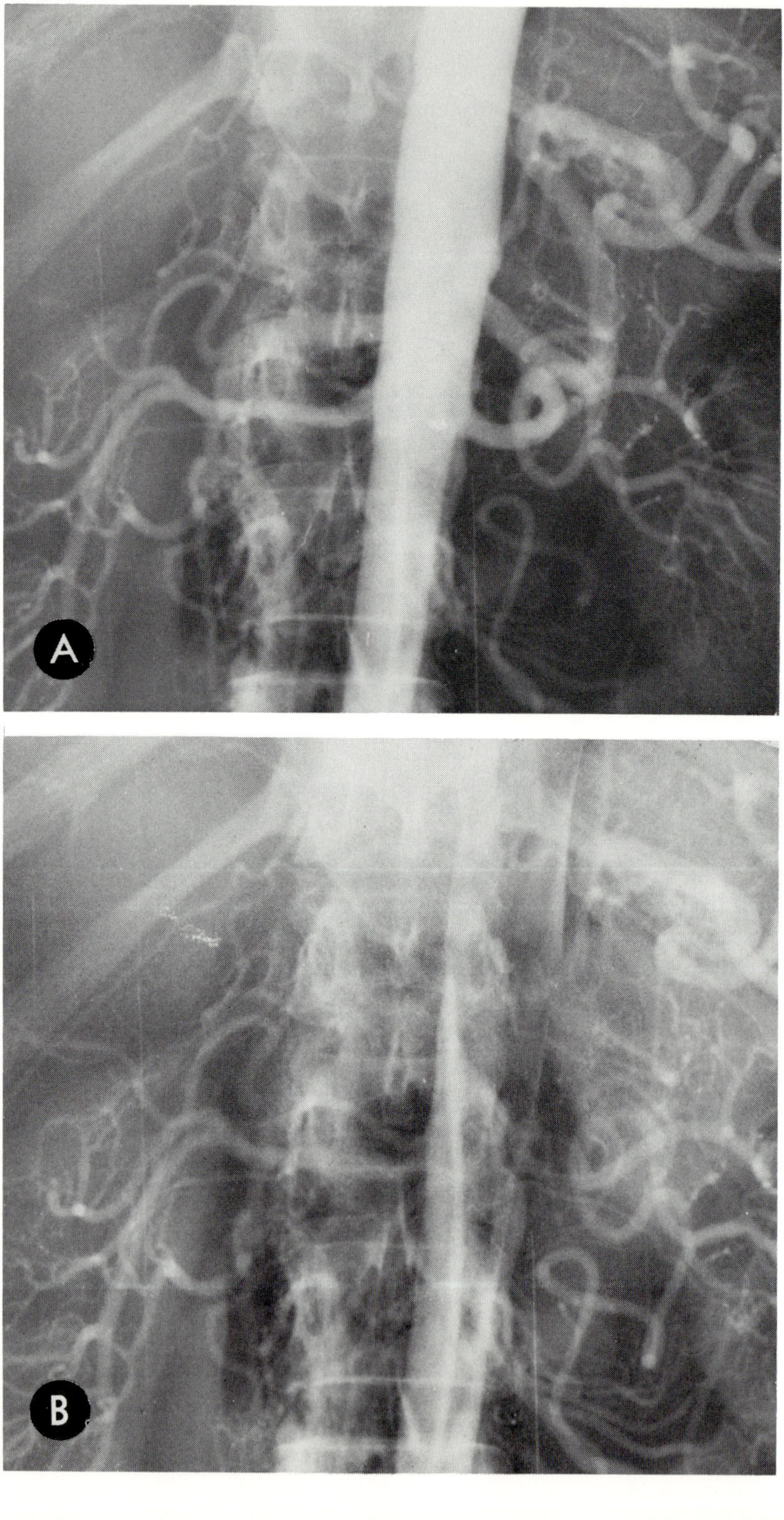
A
B

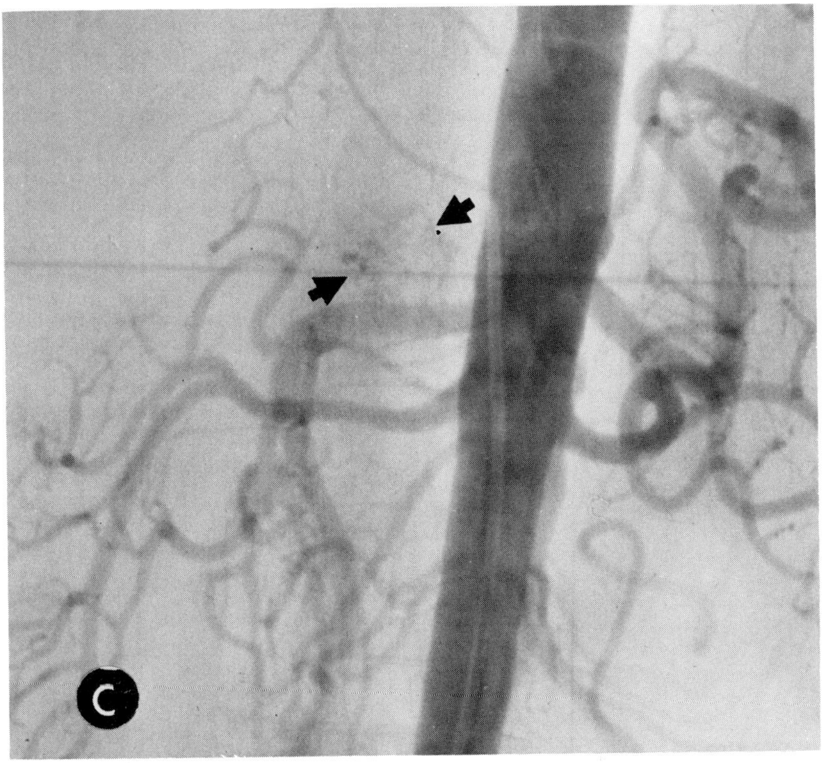

Fig. 3-5. A. Arterial phase of an anteroposterior lumbar aortogram. The main right renal artery is mildly irregular but no areas of abnormal vessels or increased contrast medium accumulation are apparent. B. Late arterial phase. No tumor vessels or other indication of a pheochromocytoma are seen. C. Subtraction film of the aortogram shown in A. A well-defined collection of abnormal vessels 2.0 cm in diameter is now apparent just above the common hepatic artery (arrows). At exploration this was a pheochromocytoma in the celiac ganglion. (Reprinted by permission from Reuter et al., ref. 82.)

20 percent of our pheochromocytoma patients undergoing arteriography it has been necessary to give small doses of phentolamine, 5 mg, to interrupt the postarteriographic hypertensive crisis. Using this approach no serious problems have resulted.

Some radiologists have suggested that the postarteriographic pressure response is so striking in patients who actually have a pheochromocytoma that the technique might be used as a diagnostic test.[76] The idea is mentioned only to help destroy it. Aside from the naiveté this view implies it reflects no awareness of potential risks inherent in arteriogra-

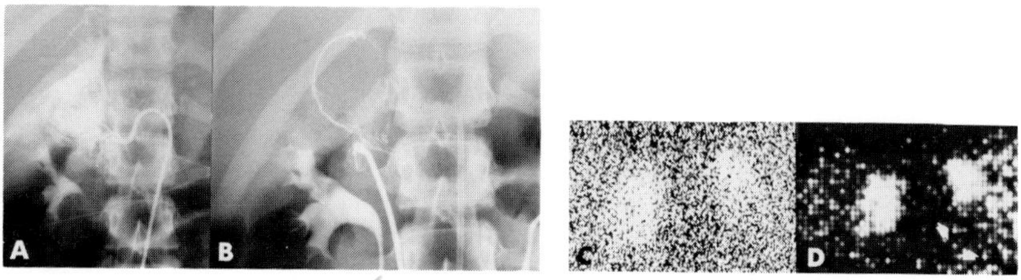

Fig. 3-6. A. Right middle adrenal arteriogram in a thirteen year female with subsequently proven right adrenal pheochromocytoma. The tumor is plainly visible in the lower aspect of the gland and the uninvolved portion of the right adrenal is displaced superiorly. B. Retrograde venogram of the same right adrenal pheochromocytoma shown in A. The magnification of this x-ray is slightly greater than in the arteriograms of A and a venous silhouette displaced by tumor mass is clearly apparent. (Courtesy of Richard P. Dorr, M.D.) C. Radiocholesterol adrenal images in the same patient. The routine scintiscan is viewed from posterior. D. Digital display of the same scintiscan. The arrows indicate decreased activity in the lower half of the right adrenal with compression of the adrenal cortex superiorly. (Reprinted by permission from Sturman et al., ref. 94.)

phy nor of the diagnostic precision available from the biochemical approaches we have already discussed.

Retrograde Adrenal Venography. A highly useful, safe and helpful radiographic technique for adrenal pheochromocytoma has been the gentle retrograde injection of angiographic dye into the venous drainage of the lesion (Fig. 3-6.). Obviously the technique requires technical refinement and skill by the angiographer. Reuter and Bookstein and various colleagues learned this technique from its originators in Sweden and England and have detailed their development of it in the United States.[81] It is useful for a variety of adrenal lesions including pheochromocytoma and the interested reader is encouraged to read their reports in detail.

When adrenal venography is used in pheochromocytoma, it is uncommon to have a severe hypertensive reaction result from the study. We have had three such reactions occur in approximately 20 venograms in patients with subsequently proven pheochromocytomas. In one patient the reaction was instigated by extravasation of the angiographic medium into a normal adrenal gland, the opposite gland harboring the tumor. Extravasation is rarely seen now in pheochromocytoma patients as technical sophistication has developed with angiography. In the other two venographic reactions the hypertensive reaction followed a well-performed venographic demonstration of the tumor. The reaction was neither marked nor prolonged. One patient required treatment with phentolamine. Sustained hypoadrenalism following retrograde venography has not occurred in our series of pheochromocytoma patients. It is seen rarely in hyperaldosteronism.

Venous Catheterization and Analysis of Regional Blood Samples for Norepinephrine and Epinephrine. In 1951, U. S. von Euler and Strom appreciated that caval catheterization with analysis of regional venous blood samples for norepinephrine and epinephrine might be helpful in localizing pheochromocytoma preoperatively. They reported a case in which the venous drainage of the tumor was accurately defined by the high content of norepinephrine draining from a lesion in the right renal hilum into the vena cava.[32] Surprisingly little use has been made of this technique in the subsequent 22 years.

The technique is simple. With local anesthesia, a tiny incision is made in the skin and a flexible radio-opaque catheter is passed through a suitably large needle into the common femoral vein. As the catheter is advanced, five blood samples are drawn, one from the vena cava just as it forms from the confluence of the common iliac veins, one just inferior to the renal veins, one from each side of the vena cava just inferior to the diaphragm and finally one in the right atrium. It is helpful if the catheter has a preformed curve at the tip. It should have a single hole near but not at the tip so that the caval blood high on the lateral aspect of the inferior vena cava superior to the adrenal venous drainage can be sampled. This will tend to reflect catecholamine input from the adrenal gland on that side. Incorrect lateralization of pheochromocytoma has occurred at the adrenal levels using this technique but this is infrequent. There is a great tendency for physicians manipulating the catheter to cannulate the adrenal vein and take samples for analysis directly from the adrenal veins. In theory this should work well because the highest catecholamine content is that which drains directly from the tumor. In fact, there is no normal range established for catecholamine content in the adrenal venous blood of human subjects under the conditions of caval catheterization. Hence, there is no rigorous standard against which increases from the pheochromocytoma might be compared. In addition, the secretory activity of the adrenal gland can be expected to vary immensely during the conditions of caval catheterization with its associated pain, uncertainty, and apprehension stimulating catecholamine release. The content of norepinephrine and epinephrine in the inferior vena cava is known, however, and forms an apt basis for comparison. Furthermore, the lower caval samples give crude standard mixed venous catecholamine content for that particular patient at

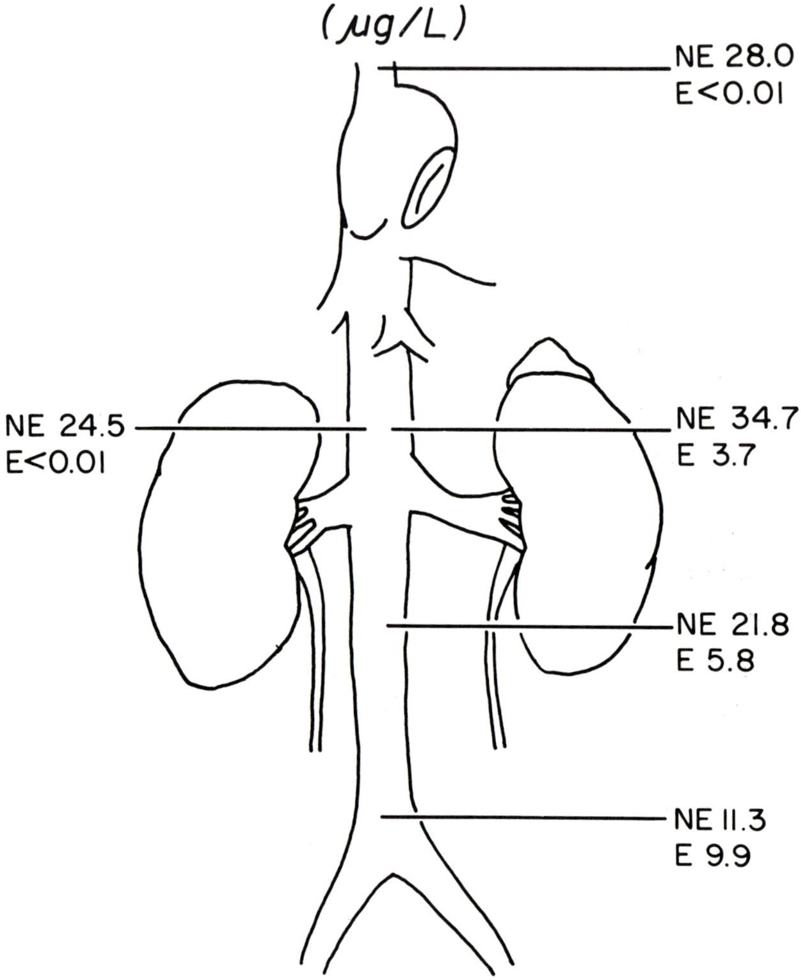

Fig. 3-7. Caval catheterization values suggesting two recurrent lesions; one near the left renal hilum and the other in the mediastinum. Both lesions were subsequently removed. The right adrenal had previously been removed for pheochromocytoma. (Reprinted by permission from Harrison and Freier, ref. 61.)

the time of the study and indicate what levels must be exceeded to suggest selective drainage of a catecholamine producing tumor into a circulation whose catecholamine levels are high already.

Caval catheterization is particularly helpful in locating small ectopically located lesions, tiny recurrences and multiple lesions too small to demonstrate any other way (Fig. 3-7). There are occasional pheochromocytoma patients who are too ill for any other procedure who have tolerated caval catheterization perfectly well.[60] Quite apart from these special situations the question arises as to when caval catheterization should be used in primary pheochromocytoma. Our feeling is that it need not be used in every case but should be used whenever there is uncertainty about the location of the pheochromocytoma. Caval catheterization is not invariably accurate, no technique is, but it is almost never misleading with respect to indicating the level of a pheochromocytoma and can give helpful information in situations in which no other technique is successful. Often it is helpful to have suggestive information from two or three localization procedures each of which may compliment and extend the validity of the other.

Photoscanning of Chromaffin Tissue. A dependably workable radioscanning technique for chromaffin tissue would be a great asset. In particular some difficult problems in recurrent pheochromocytoma could be appreciated better preoperatively than is possible at the present time.

There is no scanning technique yet available but Beierwaltes and a number of his colleagues have worked hard on this problem for almost nine years. Recently they demonstrated that [^{14}C]dopamine administered intravenously is concentrated in pheochromocytoma tissue to a sufficient degree to make imaging of the lesions feasible.[1] It now remains to label dopamine with a gamma-ray emitting isotope and there is reason to hope that this can be accomplished. Therefore there is every reason to believe that emission scanning of chromaffin tissue will become possible.

Adrenal cortical photoscanning as described by Beierwaltes and his co-workers[74] has been applied recently to the study of six patients with adrenal pheochromocytoma (Fig. 3-6). The dispersion of the adrenal cortical silhouette on the side of the pheochromocytoma has, in each case, been clear. This has given a definite negative impression of the lesion and this has been helpful.[94] Obviously this technique will not demonstrate extra-adrenal pheochromocytomas.

Surgical Removal of Pheochromocytoma

The definitive treatment of pheochromocytoma is surgical removal. As noted before, death is a well-recognized occurrence if the pheochromocytoma is not removed. Violent hypertensive and cardiovascular crisis, massive catecholamine release, and hemorrhage into a pheochromocytoma with massive catecholamine release all are known to occur and are considered far more hazardous than intelligently organized removal of the tumor.

Pheochromocytoma excision is and, no doubt, will always remain a situation requiring thoughtful collaboration between surgeon, anesthesiologist, and a cardiologically oriented internist. All three should confer and agree on the patient's preoperative care and all three should be present in the operating room at the time of pheochromocytoma excision.

Indications for preoperative adrenergic receptor blockade have been mentioned already. With respect to anesthetic premedication anticholinergic drugs such as scopolamine or atropine can be used, but cautiously since one does not wish to suddenly deprive the heart of vagal inhibition. Not infrequently a barbiturate such as Seconal or Nembutal is given in conventional doses. Occasionally, Demerol (Meperidine) has been used rather than a barbiturate. It should be recalled that Demerol is a strong vasodilator and for that reason it should be used cautiously if there is reason to believe that significant further vasodilatation might be harmful. One might, for example, hesitate to use Demerol premedication in a patient who has not had alpha adrenergic receptor blockade preoperatively.

Certain drugs should be available for immediate use in the operating room. These include norepinephine, epinephrine, phentolamine (Regitine®), propanolol, lidocaine, and hydrocortisone.

When the patient is brought to the operating room and preferably before general anesthesia is induced, a central venous pressure catheter is placed percutaneously as is a small indwelling arterial catheter. This latter is generally placed in the radial artery near the wrist. If the patient has been premedicated intelligently, he will be sleeping lightly and will tolerate the catheters gracefully if a small amount of local anesthesia is used. The central venous and arterial catheters are necessary as guides for sensitive fluid replacement and drug administration during surgery.

During the operation when cardiac dysrhythmias occur we most frequently give 1 mg of propanolol intravenously and if necessary repeat this dose twice in a 30 minute period. If this is ineffective we have rarely used an intravenous drip of lidocaine. If hypertensive bursts occur, conventional doses of 5 mg intravenous phentolamine (Regitine®) can be used. In one patient who was incompletely blocked with phenoxybenzamine 11 such doses were used in a 2 hour procedure. Some believe that preoperative phenoxybenzamine treatment prevents phentolamine from effectively reaching alpha receptors when phentolamine use is attempted during surgery.[42]

There are several opinions on what the most ideal anesthetic agent is in pheochromocytoma. We have used Innovar in approximately five patients and have found it safe and easy. Halothane is known to decrease circulating catecholamine levels and we have used this in at least a dozen of our patients. Occasional premature ventricular beats and bigeminy have been associated with Halothane but this has not been a serious problem and has responded to expeditious removal of the tumor, intravenous propanolol and in one instance intravenous lidocaine (zylocaine). A combination of Demerol and nitrous oxide has also worked well in our hands.

The operation itself need not be complicated. Exposure of the tumor can be accomplished gently with minimum manipulation of the lesion. Often the venous drainage of the tumor can be exposed, ligated, and divided before the tumor is manipulated appreciably. If the venous drainage has been demonstrated angiographically before operation, this can be a great help in locating and controlling the veins of the tumor at surgery.

On occasion it is necessary to manipulate the tumor to gain access to its venous drainage. Obviously this is a time for increased vigilance on the part of everyone for any sign of cardiovascular instability. Since the advent of selective preoperative adrenergic receptor blockade, only rarely is manipulation of the tumor associated with significant cardiovascular problems.

It should be emphasized that excessive sudden blood loss is tolerated poorly by the pheochromocytoma patient under anesthesia. Not infrequently, these lesions are closely applied to the renal veins and right-sided adrenal lesions may partially surround the inferior vena cava. With careful accurate dissection it is possible to remove the pheochromocytomas without injury to these major veins. The arterial supply to the tumor is usually diffuse and scarcely ever is a significant problem in surgical control.

If the pheochromocytoma is benign and is located in the adrenal gland it is never wise to remove the entire gland. Should a lesion develop on the opposite side, there is little excuse for the surgically induced adrenal insufficiency that would result from bilateral total adrenalectomy.

Before the advent of selective adrenergic receptor blockade, there were often critical moments associated with the tumor removal or ligation of the major veins. Such reactions of postexcision hypotension are now rare; we have not had one in the past six years. This is due to the intelligent use of adrenergic receptor blockade with coincident preoperative expansion of the plasma volume. Using the selective criteria for blockade we have mentioned previously we have not encountered postexcision hypotension in those patients in whom we have not used adrenergic receptor blockade. For this reason we feel that our criteria have selected for blockade those patients with occult or obvious contractions of their blood volume.

Rarely hypotension occurs before removal of the tumor. This is an alarming and serious problem and is most apt to occur in patients with epinephrine secreting tumors. It may represent epinephrine shock and for this reason it is well to remember that a treatment frequently effective for epinephrine shock is immediate intravenous administration of a large dose, at least 1 gm, of hydrocortisone or its equivalent if steroid analogues are used.

Some surgeons routinely inject a provocative dose of histamine or glucagon before closing the abdomen after pheochromocytoma excision. A hypertensive reaction suggests that an additional tumor may be present. One additional pheochromocytoma is alleged to have been found this way. If used at all this maneuver should never supplant careful surgical exploration of the abdominal sympathetic chains.

After the operation is over we usually keep the patient in an intensive care unit or its equivalent for 48 hours. Central venous pressure, directly recorded blood pressure from the arterial catheter, and a continuous electrocardiographic monitor are all maintained for the first 24 hours postoperatively. We remove the arterial catheter around 24 hours postoperatively and the central venous catheter about 72 hours after the operation unless there are special reasons to keep them longer.

Significant problems are seldom encountered in the late postoperative course. Discharge from the hospital is usually on or about the 8th postoperative day.

Post Surgical Follow-up

We have been in the habit of determining resting catecholamine excretion on the sixth or seventh postoperative day just prior to the patient's discharge from the hospital. Invariably there is a dramatic decrease in free catecholamine excretion at that time and unless the tumor has been unusually active, catecholamine excretion values tend to be normal by the time of discharge.

In some patients with unusually active tumors modest elevations in catecholamine excretion may persist for as long as six months post-excision. While there is no certain explanation for this, it is clear that an otherwise normal adrenergic nervous system during this time is more than normally active. This is probably an attempt to maintain, to a degree, the vascular tone to which the circulation has become accustomed in the prolonged period of catecholamine excess provided by the pheochromocytoma. In any case, it is a situation calling for reassurance rather than concern.

Following discharge the patient is followed with determination of catecholamine excretion and blood pressure at six month intervals for three years and more or less yearly thereafter. If the patient is dependable, these collections can be made at home and the samples shipped to arrive within four days for analysis. The patients can see their family physician for the follow-up visits. They should be questioned carefully for symptoms relating to recurrent hypertension and adrenergic crisis of any type.

In some patients a moderate degree of sustained hypertension may persist for as long as 2½ years postoperatively. Catecholamine excretion during this time is usually normal. The mechanism of this hypertension is not understood but many workers have noted it.[62] It is important that the patient understand that such a reacton is not unexpected, that it usually does not connote residual pheochromocytoma and that it will eventually disappear unless there is primary hypertension present from some other cause.

By far the most important reason for periodic postoperative determination of catecholamine excretion is to detect recurrent pheochromocytoma early in its course.

Recurrent Pheochromocytoma

In our experience recurrent pheochromocytoma has been a more significant problem than one might suppose from the dearth of literature available on the subject.[47,79,89] Rarely, removal of abdominal recurrence may be technically impossible.[79] Of 28 patients under our care, seven have had recurrences after a primary operation for pheochromocytoma. Of these seven, five were referred to us from the outside and two were patients whose first operation was carried out by ourselves. Hence a figure of 25 percent incidence of recurrent pheochromocytoma is undoubtedly greatly weighted in a referral center with an interest in the disease. On the other hand, the problem occurs not infrequently, at least 10 percent of the time, and is considerably more complex than primary pheochromocytoma. For these reasons recurrent pheochromocytoma merits special attention.

Recurrent pheochromocytoma is best understood from the perspective of the precise pathology represented in the individual recurrence. All of these patients manifest symptoms of excessive catecholamine release and excretion. While it is theoretically possible that nonfunctioning recurrences of a primary functioning chromaffin cell tumor might occur, we have not encountered this phenomenon either in our experience or in our review of the literature.

Roughly 10 percent of primary pheochromocytoma patients harbor multiple benign lesions. Most, but not all, of these multiple primaries are obvious at the time of the first exploration. Occasionally second and third benign primary lesions occur after the first has been removed. One patient under our care, a boy of 10, had a recurrence become apparent from hypertensive attacks, the first of which occurred $1\frac{1}{2}$ years after an initial pheochromocytoma was removed from the right adrenal gland. Both the second and third pheochromocytomas were apparent at the time of the second operation. One was located in the sympathetic chain of the right superior mediastinum and was visible on routine chest x-ray.[61] The other was located in the left lumbar sympathetic chain in close proximity to the left renal vein and artery. Both of these lesions were obvious on caval catheterization (Fig. 3-7) and that in the left renal hilum could not be demonstrated by any other means. The left perihilar renal lesion was the more active as judged from the caval catheterization studies and was removed first. At a third operation ten days later the mediastinal lesion was removed through a right posterolateral thoracotomy. Adrenergic receptor blockade had been used prior to the second operation and was instituted four days afterwards in preparation for the third operation. Staging of these two pheochromocytoma excisions was perfectly smooth and preferable, in our opinion, to attempting removal of both lesions at one operation.

A second type of recurrence is located near the site of removal of the primary lesion. Such a lesion is shown arteriographically in Figure 3-8. Surgical removal of this lesion was simple and the recurrence was independent of the urinary bladder although this had not been true of the primary.[51] We regard this as a benign recurrence since there were no other abdominal lesions associated with it, six of six pelvic lymph nodes examined were free of tumor, and the patient's catecholamine excretion has been normal for 6 years since the recurrence was removed.

A third patient experienced recurrent pheochromocytoma in conjunction with her second pregnancy, 12 years following removal of a right sided infrarenal primary pheochromocytoma. Her recurrences were four in number, neighboring and overlying the junction of the vena cava and the right renal vein.[69] One recurrence was located adjacent to lymph node tissue microscopically but is probably not a malignant recurrence. Excision of these four nodules has given this patient eight asymptomatic years and she is doing well at the present time.

A 12-year-old boy had clear biochemical evidence of a recurrent

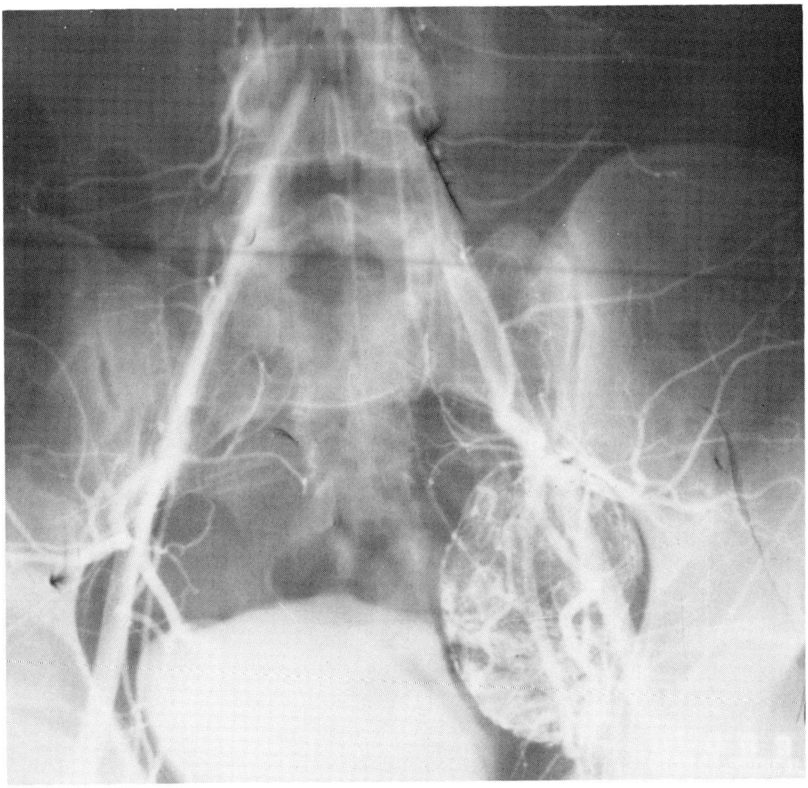

Fig. 3-8. A large recurrence of a bladder pheochromocytoma is demonstrated arteriographically in proximity to the bladder. The patient is asymptomatic and has normal catecholamine excretion rates seven years after excision of this recurrence. (Reprinted by permission from Harrison et al., ref. 51.)

pheochromocytoma. Two adrenal pheochromocytomas had been removed $1\frac{1}{2}$ years previously. Caval catheterization could not be performed on this second admission because the necessary laboratory equipment and personnel were being moved to another country. At a thorough abdominal exploration, no recurrent abdominal disease could be found. We think it is likely that his lesion is ectopically located, perhaps in the mediastinum. Undoubtedly caval catheterization would have been immensely helpful in locating his recurrence which could be a third primary pheochromocytoma. The issue is not yet resolved and the patient is still asymptomatic.[53]

A 53-year-old male underwent removal of a primary pheochromocytoma of the left adrenal gland 21 years before referral to us for recurrent debilitating attacks of hypertension, palpitations and extreme anxiety. For seven years prior to his admission even the most delicate Val Salva maneuver elicited a hypertensive crisis. His lesion secreted a mixture of norepinephrine and epinephrine. Caval catheterization demonstrated catecholamine input at the left renal hilar level. An abdominal exploration of three and one half hours was technically difficult. On a third frozen section of extensive chronic retroperitoneal fat necrosis, diffusely microscopic recurrences of pheochromocytoma cells were found. This is a unique example of this type of recurrent pheochromocytoma. Total excision of this tissue was technically impossible. That patient had a prolonged stormy course complicated by pulmonary and abdominal sepsis and recurrent problems related to excessive circulating catecholamines. He died on the 106th postoperative day. Postmortem exam showed miliary pulmonary metastases. A preoperative chest x-ray was normal.

Two other patients developed widespread metastases from malignant pheochromocytoma and will be discussed later.

From these clinical vignettes, several important points concerning recurrent pheochromocytoma can be made. One is that an aggressive surgical approach to recurrent pheochromocytoma can yield gratifying long term palliation and cure. Secondly caval catheterization is indispensable in understanding the type and location of the recurrences. Thirdly, diffuse microscopic recurrence of pheochromocytoma is possible and may frustrate efficient understanding of the nature of the problem at surgery. Finally, if it is not possible to remove a substantial part of the recurrent pheochromocytoma, a stormy postoperative course characteristic of continually excessive catecholamine release is likely to occur.

Malignant Pheochromocytoma

It is commonly stated that approximately 10 percent of pheochromocytomas are malignant and in our experience of three malignancies in 28 patients, this has proven to be true. As with many endocrine neoplasms cellular morphology is not dependable for establishing malignancy. The only certain criterion for malignancy in pheochromocytoma is the demonstration of viable chromaffin cells in locations where chromaffin cells customarily do not occur. Examples of such sites are lymph nodes, liver and lungs.

Malignant pheochromocytomas are able to synthesize norepinephrine from its precursors, a fact confirmed by a number of independent investigators.[3,83] Evidently the rate-limiting feedback inhibition of tyrosine hydroxylase by norepinephrine and epinephrine does not take place effectively in malignant pheochromocytoma. The high levels of circulating catecholamines certainly do nothing to limit increased urinary catecholamine or catecholamine metabolite excretion and the picture is one of autonomous unrestrained continual release of catecholamines. There is evidence to suggest that conversion of norepinephrine to epinephrine in malignant pheochromocytoma requires large quantities of adrenal cortical hormones just as it does physiologically. Kennedy et al. analyzed a primary adrenal pheochromocytoma at postmortem examination which contained abundant norepinephrine and epinephrine. Hepatic metastases contained only norepinephrine.[70]

It is important to realize that an aggressive attitude toward pheochromocytoma recurrences including focal malignant recurrences can yield gratifying long-term palliation. Surgery for widespread functioning metastases in pheochromocytoma is foolish, however, since there are undoubtedly many lesions beyond the limits of judicious surgical removal.

As previously noted, an effective chromaffin cell scan would be immensely helpful in demonstrating occult miliary spread of pheochromocytoma and conceivably could be used to deliver therapeutic radiation to the same lesions.

Considerable effort has been expended in recent years in developing effective palliation of the symptoms associated with chronic catecholamine excess in malignant pheochromocytoma. Great hopes were attached to pharmacologic inhibition of tyrosine hydroxylase. Of a large number of drugs tested the most suitable inhibitor of this enzyme for clinical use proved to be alpha methyl-paratyrosine. Administration of this agent to patients with functioning metastatic pheochromocytoma does, in fact, result in approximately 60 percent reduction in free catecholamine excretion and significant blunting of the patient's symptoms.[87] Unfortunately, therapeutic levels of alpha methyl-paratyrosine may damage the kidneys and are associated with side effects of severe nausea, anorexia and weakness which some patients find disagreeable.

In our experience chronic partial adrenergic receptor blockade with orally administered phenoxybenzamine and propanolol when indicated has worked much better for palliation of symptomatic malignant pheochromocytoma. One patient with norepinephrine secreting lesions who could not tolerate alpha methyl-paratyrosine has now been managed successfully for six years on low doses of phenoxybenzamine, 20 mg tid by mouth, and oral propanolol, 15 mg tid. Postural hypotension has not been a problem at this dosage level and the patient has had good palliation of hypertensive attacks which previously kept him inactive. Currently this patient is able to work full time as a waiter and bus boy.

Occasionally he takes an extra dose of both drugs if he feels an attack coming on but has never had to use an extra dose more than once in a given day and most frequently does not have to do so at all. His current free norepinephrine excretion rate of 347 μg per 24 hours is well tolerated. He is thought to have miliary pulmonary metastases on chest x-ray in addition to recognized abdominal recurrences in the liver and lymph nodes.

A 36-year-old housewife was referred to us with recurrent symptoms after reexploration for recurrent tumor had been negative. She had a stormy postoperative course following her second exploration. Her primary left adrenal epinephrine secreting lesion had been removed five years before. Caval catheterization of this patient was unconvincing at any level showing a generalized symmetrical increase in all samples, but the highest was from the bed of the left adrenal. A chest x-ray was negative. Abdominal exploration was negative. Following this third operation, the patient had a stormy postoperative course complicated by staphylococcal pneumonia of the right lower lobe. Every time the right lobe was suctioned with a catheter, she had a hypertensive crisis. After her discharge, she was managed successfully with oral regitine taking it three times daily and supplementing it with an extra dose whenever she felt an attack coming on. She was able to lead an active life this way but wished to have further surgery.

Repeat caval catheterization was again suggestive but ambiguous. Another chest film was negative. The patient did not receive adrenergic receptor blockade before any of her operations including this fourth one and at the end of a fruitless 3 hour operation she became hypotensive with mild pulmonary edema. It was not possible to restore an effective blood pressure. At postmortem examination macroscopic pulmonary metastases were found in the superior segment of the right lower lobe and diffuse microscopic spread was apparent throughout the right lung.[51] It was this patient that first demonstrated to us the need for routine beta and alpha adrenergic receptor blockade in predominantly epinephrine secreting tumors. Had we catheterized the left side of the heart, particularly the right pulmonary vein, we could have had evidence of the pulmonary lesion which was not visualized on x-ray. This is a bizarre clinical situation and is useful in emphasizing the point that recurrent pheochromocytoma is, frequently, a bizarre and unique situation pathologically and requires more than conventional understanding.

Isolated attempts have been made at x-radiation of malignant pheochromocytoma as well as with the use of antimetabolic drugs for disseminated pheochromocytoma. These efforts have met with so little improvement in the patient's condition that x-ray and tumor chemotherapy are generally not resorted to in current day palliation of malignant pheochromocytoma. It is, however, not illogical to hope that specific chemotherapy or specific radiation therapy directed to the malignant cells synthesizing catecholamines might become possible in the near future by well-tolerated agents which effectively inhibit the biosynthesis of catecholamines.

Other Catecholamine Synthesizing Tumors

Although not, in the conventional sense, among surgical disorders of the mature adrenal gland other catecholamine synthesizing tumors should be mentioned. Prominent among these is neuroblastoma, an aggressively malignant neoplasm of childhood, arising from undifferentiated adrenal and/or ectopically located pheochromoblasts. This tumor is biochemically visible, so to speak, by virtue of the excretion of increased quantities of one or another of one or another of the catecholamine precursors and their metabolites.[19] Not uncommonly the biosynthesis is carried all the way to norepinephrine but even when that is accomplished it is done so in a biochemically inefficient way as indicated by the finding of increased quantities of precursors and their metabolites in the urine. Aggressive surgical treatment and radiation therapy may occasionally cure neuroblastoma. The most sensitive indication of early recurrence of the tumor is demonstration of increased excretion of the same metabolites or catecholamines whose increased excretion was demonstrated initially. Thus, if one is confronted with a child whose homovanillic acid excretion rate is again elevated after becoming normal following the excision of a primary tumor, abdominal re-exploration and if feasible, excision of recurrent tumor is indicated on that basis alone. If a tumor cannot be resected, it can at least be outlined with metallic clips to help guide future x-ray therapy. Various protocols combining anti-tumor chemotherapy and radiation therapy in neuroblastoma are being studied and are currently in progress in several centers dealing with malignant diseases of children. Perhaps something substantive will come from these efforts.

Uncommonly ganglioneuromas and chemodectomas may synthesize catecholamines probably from lesions arising from chromaffin cells within these structures. LeCompte has worked hard to make a case for nonchromaffin cell tumors of the carotid bodies synthesizing catecholamines but most of this evidence was developed before modern precision in catecholamine analysis was achieved. Interested readers are advised to study LeCompte's work[72] and form their own opinion.

Rarely patients with tumors secreting large quantities of dopamine present with profound and relenteless diarrhea. This subsides with removal of tumor.[41] If diarrhea occurs in connection with functioning metastases, attempts should be made to control the symptoms with partial adrenergic receptor blockade if the recurrent tumor cannot be excised. It is frequently a difficult matter to palliate diarrhea successfully, however, and if partial adrenergic receptor blockade does not work, it is worthwhile to attempt palliation with tyrosine hydroxylase inhibitors.

REFERENCES

1. Anderson BG, Beierwaltes WH, Harrison TS, Ansari AN, Buswick AA: Labelled dopamine concentration in pheochromocytoma. J Nuc Med 14:781, 1973
2. Angell-James JE, deBurgh Daly M: Comparison of the reflex Vasomotor responses to separate and combined stimulation of the carotid sinus and aortic arch barorecptors by pulsatile and non-pulsatile pressures in the dog. J Physiol 209:257, 1970
3. Anton A, Greer M, Sayre DF, Williams CM: Dihydroxyphenylalanine secretion in a malignant pheochromocytoma. Amer J Med 42:469, 1967
4. Axelrod J: *O*-Methylation of epinephrine and other catecholamines in vitro and in vivo. Science 126:400, 1957
5. Axelrod J: Metabolism of epinephrine and other sympathomimetic amines. Physiol Rev 39:751, 1959
6. Axelrod J, Weinshilboum R: Catecholamines. NEJM 287:237, 1972
7. Axelrod J, Weil-Malherbe H, Tomchick R: The physiological disposition of ^{3}H-epinephrine and its metabolite metanephrine. J Pharmacol Exp Ther 127:251, 1959
8. Birke G, Duner H, Liljedahl SO, Pernow B, Plantin LO, Turell L: Histamine, catecholamine and adrenocortical steroids in burns. Acta Chir Scand 114:87, 1957
9. Blaschko HC: The specific action of L-dopa decarboxylase. J Physiol 96:50P, 1939
10. Blaschko HC: The activity of L(−)-dopa decarboxylase. J Physiol 101:337, 1942
11. Bogaert MG, Vermuelen A: Pheochromocytoma of the urinary bladder with inconclusive chemical and pharmacologic tests. Amer J Med 53:797, 1972
12. Brown GL, Gillespie JF: The output of sympathetic transmitter from the spleen of the cat. J Physiol 138:81, 1957
13. Burn JH, Rand MJ: Sympathetic postganglionic mechanism. Nature 184:163, 1959

14. Burn H, Rand MJ: Sympathetic postganglionic cholinergic fibers. Brit J Pharmacol Chemother 15:56, 1960
15. Burn JH, Rand MJ: Acetylcholine in adrenergic transmission. Ann Rev Pharmacol 5:163, 1965
16. Caldwell FT, Osterholm JC, Sower ND, Moyer CA: Metabolic response to thermal trauma of normal and thyroprivic rats at three environmental temperatures. Ann Surg 150:976, 1959
17. Cannon WB, McIver MA, Bliss SW: A sympathetic and adrenal mechanism for mobilizing sugar in hypoglycemia. Am J Physiol 69:46, 1924
18. Christensen NJ: Increased levels of plasma noradrenaline in hypothyroidism. J Clin Endocrinol Metab 35:359, 1972
19. Chatten J, Voorhess ML: Familial neuroblastoma. NEJM 277:1230, 1967
20. Clarke DD, Wilk S, Gitlow SE, et al.: Gas chromotographic determination of dopamine at the nanogram level. J Gas Chromatog 5:307, 1967
21. Coden J: Pheochromocytoma in pregnancy. Proc Roy Soc Med Eng 65:863, 1972
22. Cope O, Nardi G, Quijano M, Rovit RL, Stanbury JB, Wight A: Metabolic rate and thyroid function following acute thermal trauma in man. Ann Surg 137:165, 1953
23. Duner H: The influence of the blood glucose level on the secretion of adrenaline and noradrenaline from the suprarenal. Acta Phys Scand 28:Suppl. 102, 1953
24. Egdahl RH, Chobanian AN: Acute pheochromocytoma. Surg Clin N Amer 46:645, 1966
25. Engelman F, Portnoy B: A sensitive double-isotope derivative assay for norepinephrine and epinephrine: normal resting human plasma levels. Circ Res 26:53, 1970
26. Euler US von: The presence of a substance with sympathin-E properties in spleen extracts. Acta Phys Scand 11:168, 1946a
27. Euler US von: A specific sympathetic sympathomimetic ergone in adrenergic fibers (sympathin) and its relation to adrenaline and noradrenaline. Acta Phys Scand 12:73, 1946b
28. Euler US von: Identification of the sympathomimetic ergone in adrenergic nerves of cattle (sympathin N) with laevo-noradrenaline. Acta Phys Scand 16:63, 1948
29. Euler US von, Folkow B: Selective activation of noradrenaline and adrenaline producing cells in the suprarenal gland of the cat by hypothalamic stimulation. Circ Res 2:191, 1954
30. Euler US von, Lishajko F: Improved technique for fluorometric estimation of catecholamines. Acta Phys Scand 51:348, 1961
31. Euler US von, Luft R, Sundin T: The urinary excretion of noradrenaline and adrenaline in healthy subjects during recumbency and standing. Acta Phys Scand 34:169, 1955

32. Euler, US von, et al.: Report of a case of pheochromocytoma with special regard to preoperative diagnostic problems. Acta Med Scand 153:127, 1955
33. Flint JM: The blood vessels, angiogenesis, organogenesis, reticulum and histology of the adrenal. The Johns Hopkins Hospital Reports 9:153, 1900
34. Folkow B, Euler US von: op cit Ref. 28
35. Frankenheuser M, Mellis J, Rissler A, et al.: Catecholamine excretion as related to cognitive and emotional reaction patterns. Psychosom Med 30:109, 1968
36. Franksson C, Gemzell CA, Euler US von: Cortical and medullary adrenal activity in surgical and allied conditions. J Clin Endocrinol 14:608, 1954
37. Freier DT, Harrison, TS: Rigorous biochemical criteria for the diagnosis of pheochromocytoma. J Surg Res 14:177, 1973
38. Funk C: Synthesis of *d,l*-3:4-dihydroxyphenylalanine. J Chem Soc 99:554, 1911
39. Goodall MCC, Alton H: Dopamine (3-hydroxytyramine) replacement and metabolism in sympathetic nerve and adrenal medullary depletions after prolonged thermal injury. J Clin Invest 48:1761, 1969
40. Goodall McC, Stone C, Haynes BW: Urinary output of adrenaline and noradrenaline in severe thermal burns. Ann Surg 145:479, 1957
41. Greenberg RE, Gardner LI: Catecholamine metabolism in a functioning neural tumor. J Clin Invest 39:1729, 1960
42. Gupta S, Ternberg JL, Weldon VV, Pagliara AS: Alpha adrenergic blocking agent in childhood pheochromocytoma. Surgery 74:551, 1973
43. Hammond WG, Arnow L, Moore FR: Studies in surgical endocrinology III. Ann Surg 144:715, 1956
44. Harrison TS: Reflex liberation of catecholamines in hyperthyroidism. J Surg Res 1:77, 1961
45. Harrison TS: Adrenaline and noradrenaline excretion following burns. J Trauma 7:137, 1967
46. Harrison TS: Adrenal medullary and thyroid relationships. Physiol Rev 44:161, 1964
47. Harrison TS, Freier DT: Recurrent pheochromocytoma. Arch Surg 108:450–454, 1974
48. Harrison TS, Seaton JF: Respiratory influences on the secretion of catecholamines. J Surg Res 5:556, 1965
49. Harrison TS, Seaton JF: The relative effects of hypoxia and hypercarbia on adrenal medullary secretion in anesthetized dogs. J Surg Res 5:560, 1965
50. Harrison TS, Bartlett JD Jr, Seaton JF: Exaggerated urinary norepinephrine response to tilt in pheochromocytoma. NEJM 277:725, 1967
51. Harrison TS, Bartlett JD Jr, Seaton JF: Current evaluation and management of pheochromocytoma. Ann Surg 168:701, 1968
52. Harrison TS, Bartlett JD Jr, Seaton JF: Adrenal medulla: some

basic and clinical considerations with special reference to pheochromocytoma; in cardiac and vascular diseases. H. Conn and O. Hurwitz, (eds), Lea & Febiger, Phila., 1971, 1735 pgs
53. Harrison TS, Birbari A, Seaton JF: Malignant hypertension in pheochromocytoma: correlation with plasma renin activity. Johns Hopkins Med J 130:329, 1972
54. Harrison TS, Chawla RC, Seaton JF, Robinson BH: Carotid sinus origin of adrenergic responses compromising the effectiveness of artificial circulatory support. Surgery 68:20, 1970
55. Harrison TS, Birbari A, Seaton JF: Reinforcement of reflex epinephrine release by angiotensin II. Am J Phys 224:31, 1973
56. Harrison TS, Seaton JF, Bartlett JD Jr.: Adrenergic mechanisms in acute hypovolemia. Surg Forum 17:66, 1966
57. Harrison TS, Dagher FJ, Beck L, Bartlett JD Jr: Rationale and indications for preoperative adrenergic receptor blockade in pheochromocytoma. Med Clin N Amer 53:1349, 1969
58. Harrison TS, Seaton JF, Feller I: Relationship of increased oxygen consumption to catecholamine excretion in thermal burns. Ann Surg 165:169, 1967
59. Harrison TS, Silver DM, Zuidema GD: Thyroid and adrenal medullary function in chronic executive monkeys. Endocrinology 78:685, 1966
60. Harrison TS, Seaton JF, Cerny JC, Bookstein JJ, Bartlett JD Jr: Localization of pheochromocytoma by caval catheterization. Arch Surg 95:339, 1967
61. Harrison TS, Freier DT: Pitfalls in the technique and interpretation of regional venous sampling for localizing pheochromocytoma. Surg Clin N Am 54:339, 1974
62. Herrman H, Mornex R: Human tumors secreting catecholamines. Pergamon Press, The Macmillan Company, NY, 1964
63. Hillarp NA, Hokfelt B: Evidence of adrenaline and noradrenaline in separate adrenal medullary cells. Acta Physiol Scand 30:55, 1953
64. Hökfelt T, Fuxe K, Goldstein M, Joh TN: Immunohistochemical localization of three catecholamine synthesizing enzymes. Histochemie 33:231, 1973
65. Hökfelt T, Fuxe K, Goldstein M: Immunohistochemical studies on monamine-containing cell systems. Brain Res 62:461, 1973
66. Hume DM: Pheochromocytoma in adult and child. Amer J Surg 99:458, 1960
67. Iversen LL: Uptake of catecholamines at high perfusion concentration in rat isolated heart: a novel catecholamine uptake process. Brit J Pharmacol 25:18, 1965
68. Iversen LL: The uptake and storage of noradrenaline in sympathetic nerves. Cambridge University Press, London and New York, 1967, 253
69. Jaffe RB, Harrison TS, Cerny JC: Localization of metastatic pheo-

chromocytoma in pregnancy by caval catheterization and including urinary catecholamine values of uncomplicated pregnancies. Am J Obstet Gynec 104:939, 1969

70. Kennedy JS, Symington T, Woodger BA: Chemical and histochemical observations in benign and malignant pheochromocytoma. J Path Bact 81:409, 1961
71. Leak D, Brunjes S: Adrenal medullary secretion in hyperthyroidism. Lancet 1:863, April 21, 1962
72. LeCompte PM: Tumors of the carotid body and related structures. Atlas of tumor pathology, Fasc. 16, Washington, D.C., Armed Forces Institute of Pathology, 1951
73. Leduc J: Catecholamine production and release in exposure and acclimation to cold. Acta Physiol Scand 53:Suppl. 183, 1961
74. Lieberman LM, Beierwaltes WH, Conn JW, et al.: Diagnosis of adrenal diseases by visualization of human adrenal glands with ^{131}I-19-iodocholesterol. NEJM 285:1387, 1971
75. Maebashi M, Miura Y, Yoshinage K: Plasma renin activity in pheochromocytoma. Jap Circ J 32:1427, 1968
76. Meaney TF, Buonocore E: Selective arteriography as a localizing and provocative test in the diagnosis of pheochromocytoma. Radiology 87:309, 1966
77. Morris ME, Millar RA: Blood pH/plasma catecholamine relationships: non-respiratory acidosis. Brit J Anesthesiol 34:682, 1962
78. Mornex R, Fitoussi R, Pousset G, Perrin N: Effects d'un moderateur du systeme sympathique en pathologie thyroidienne. La Revue Lyonnaise de Medecine 18:71, 1969
79. Pinet A, Mornex R, Perrin J, Minh VT, Veyret C: Pheochromocytome de la concavite sacree erodant le sacrom et los iliaque. J Radio Electrol 53:851, 1972
80. Priestly JT, Kvale, WF, Gifford, RW: Pheochromytoma. Arch Surg 86:778, 1963
81. Reuter SR, Blair AJ, Schteingart DE, Bookstein JJ: Adrenal venography. 89:805, 1967
82. Reuter SR, Talner LB, Atkin T: The importance of subtraction in the angiographic evaluation of extra-adrenal pheochromocytomas, Am J Roentgenol 117:128, 1973
83. Robinson R, Smith P, Whittaker SRF: Secretion of catecholamine in malignant pheochromocytoma. Brit Med J 1:1422, 1964
84. Scott HW, Riddell DH, Brockman SR: Surgical management of pheochromocytoma. Surg Gynec Obstet 120:707, 1965
85. Sellwood RA, Wapnick S, Breckenride A, Williams ED, Welburn RB: Recurrent pheochromocytoma. Brit J Surg 57:309, 1970
86. Silver DM, Seaton JF, Harrison TS: Adrenal epinephrine and norepinephrine content following denervation and barbiturates. J Surg Res 8:177, 1968
87. Sjoerdsma A, Engelman K, Spector S, Udenfriend S: Inhibition of

catecholamine synthesis in man with alpha methyl-para-tyrosine, an inhibitor of tyrosine hydroxylase. Lancet 2:1092, 1965

88. Steinman AM, Smerin SE, Barchas JD: Epinephrine metabolism in mammalian brain after intravenous and intraventricular administration. Science 165:616, 1969
89. Sjoerdsma A, England K, Waldman TA, Cooperman LH, Hammond WG: Pheochromocytoma: current concepts of diagnosis and treatment. Ann Int Med 65:1302, 1966
90. Stoffer SS, Jiang N, Gorman CA, Pikler GM: Plasma catecholamines in hypothyroidism and hyperthyroidism. J Clin Endocrinol Metab 36:587, 1973
91. Studnitz W von: Chemistry and pharmacology of catecholamine producing tumors. Pharmacol Rev 18:645, 1966
92. Studnitz W von: Provokationstests beim Phäochromozytom. Deutsch Med Wochenschr 95:1934, 1970
93. Studnitz W von: Glukagontest und Phaochromozytomdiagnostik. Schweiz Med Wschr 100:1023, 1970
94. Sturman MF, Moses DC, Beierwaltes WH, Harrison TS, Ice RD, Dorr RP: Radiocholesterol adrenal imaging in the localization of pheochromocytoma. Surg Gynec Obstet 138:177, 1974
95. Taniguchi J, Kakimoto Y, Armstrong MD: Quantitative determination of metanephrine and normetanephrine in urine. J Lab Clin Med 64:469, 1964
96. Van Way CW III, Michaelakis AM, Alper B, et al.: Renal vein renin studies in a patient with renal hilar pheochromocytoma and renal artery stenosis. Ann Surg 172:212, 1970
97. Werning C, et al.: Die Plasma-Renin-Aktivität beim Phädochromozytom. Deutsch Med Wschr, 95:117, 1970
98. Wurtman RJ, Axelrod J: Control of enzymatic synthesis of adrenaline in the adrenal medulla by adrenal cortical steroids. J Biol Chem 241:2301, 1966
99. Wilmore DW, Long JM, Mason AD Jr, et al.: Catecholamines: mediator of the hypermetabolic response to thermal trauma. Ann Surg, 180:653, 1974

4

Surgical Approaches to the Adrenal Gland

POSTERIOR APPROACH TO ADRENALECTOMY

The primary indications for bilateral total adrenalectomy are Cushing's disease, "idiopathic" hyperaldosteronism, and palliation for metastatic carcinoma of the breast. Unilateral adrenalectomy is performed for tumors of the adrenal cortex and medulla.

Over the years, a number of different surgical approaches to the adrenal glands have been devised; anterior (transabdominal), posterior, transthoracic, and lumbar approaches have all had their various proponents. Nowadays, however, most contemporary surgeons favor either the posterior or the anterior approach.

The anterior approach is indicated in pheochromocytoma, when it is necessary to examine the entire abdominal cavity so as to rule out the presence of ectopic or metastatic tumor. The anterior approach is also used when an adrenocortical carcinoma is suspected; it provides the wide exposure needed to resect the tumor en bloc.

In most other situations, however, the posterior approach is preferred. From the posterior approach, the adrenal glands are more superficially located than is generally realized, and they can be exposed directly without the need for extensive mobilization or retraction of adjacent viscera. Consequently, prolonged post operative ileus is rarely a problem and the chance for inadvertant visceral injury is less. Use of the posterior approach to perform adrenalectomy has substantially reduced the morbidity associated with the procedure.

Crile[3] first used the posterior exposure to perform adrenal denervation as a treatment for hypertension and his technique was later adapted by Young[9] for adrenalectomy. It was Smithwick[8] from Boston University Hospital who emphasized that the key to the operation is removal of the 12th rib; he pointed out that with the underlying pleura reflected upwards out of harm's way, and the diaphragm divided, the exposure of the adrenal is excellent.

The Operation

After induction of anesthesia and insertion of an endotracheal tube, the patient is positioned face-downward on the table. Great care should be exercised when turning the patient who has metastatic breast cancer if the cervical spine is the seat of advanced disease. Hemiplegia can be produced by vertebral collapse and spinal compression during this change in position.[1]

Rolls are placed beneath the chest and pelvis. The abdomen sags between them and the intra-abdominal organs fall away from the retroperitoneal space. The diaphragm is thereby allowed free excursion—a factor which undoubtedly contributes to the low incidence of postoperative pulmonary complications in these patients. The operating table is flexed into the jack-knife position to eliminate most of the lumbar lordosis and the patient's legs are supported on two large pillows to circumvent venous pooling in the calves (Fig. 4-1).

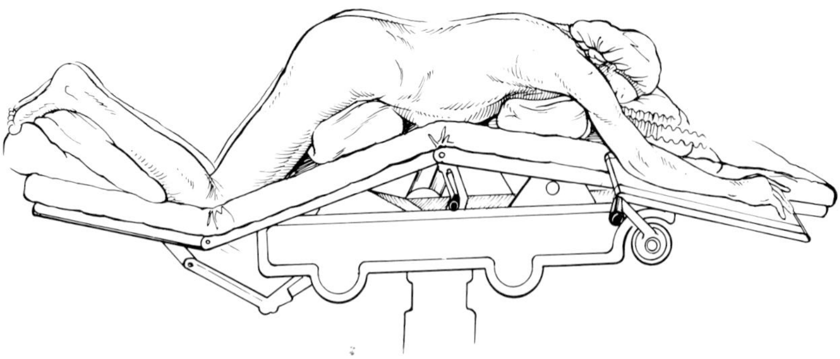

Fig. 4-1. Shown is the patient's position used for the posterior approach to the adrenal glands.

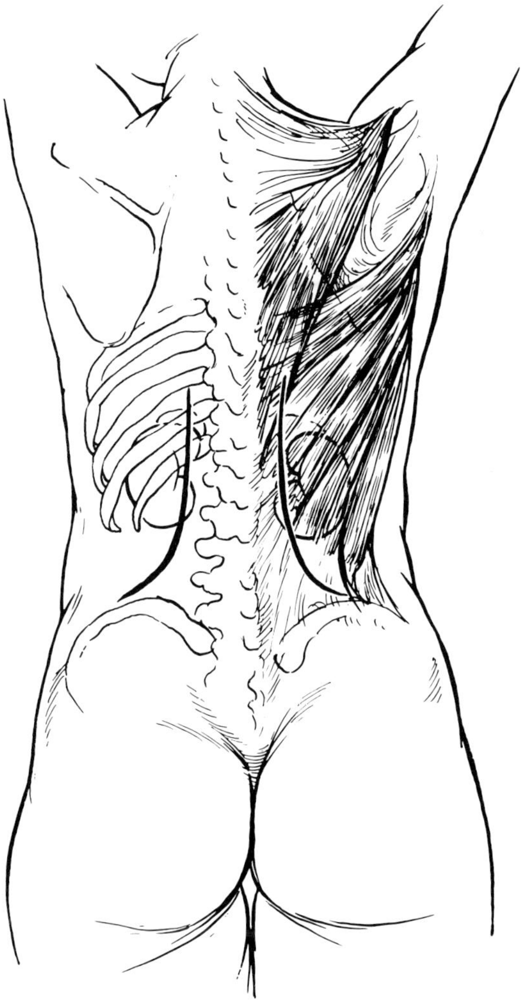

Fig. 4-2. Incisions for the bilateral approach to the adrenals are shown.

The skin incision is made beginning about 3 fingerbreadths from the midline at the level of the 10th rib. From there, it is directed obliquely downward and outward taking a gentle curve to meet the iliac crest at a point about 4 fingerbreadths from the midline. When bilateral adrenalectomy is planned, two operating teams can work simultaneously on opposite sides of the table (Fig. 4-2). We will describe removal of the right adrenal. Important variations for the left side will be mentioned.

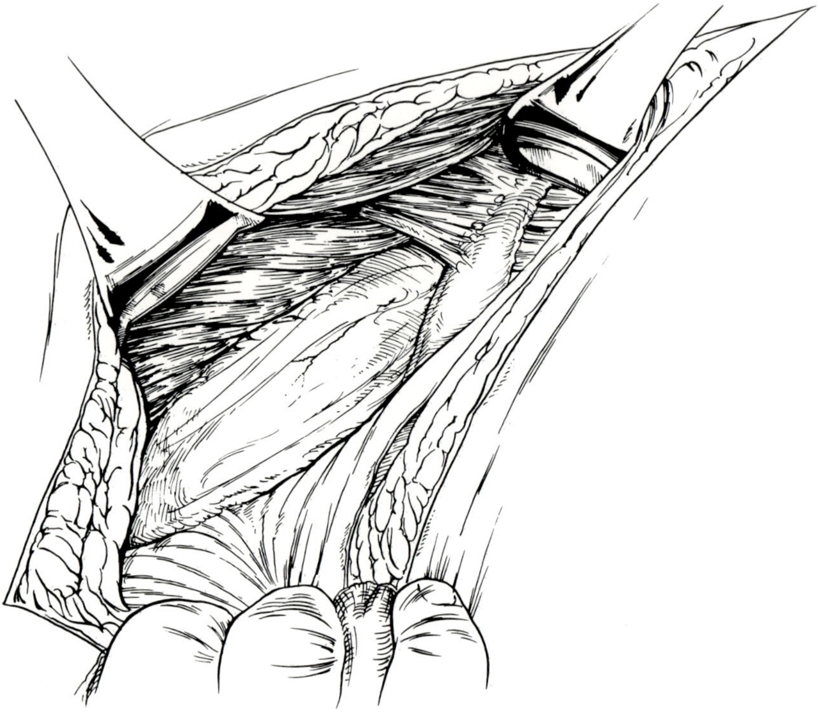

Fig. 4-3. Exposure of the right twelfth rib using the posterior skin incision on the right, shown in Figure 4-2.

The incision is carried down through the subcutaneous fat, the latissimus dorsi and the posterior lamella of the lumbodorsal fascia. The sacrospinalis is then retracted medially and its pedicle attachment to the 12th rib severed. Several small, constant bleeders, branches of the last intercostal and lumbar vessels emerging from the muscle, may have to be individually clamped and ligated (Fig. 4-3).

The 12th rib is removed subperiosteally, care being taken to avoid the underlying pleura (Fig. 4-4).

The leash of intercostal vessels are exposed by removal of the rib; they are divided between clamps and ligated. The subcostal nerve which lies at a somewhat deeper plane, is preserved and retracted inferiorly out of harm's way.

The conjoined middle and anterior lamellae of the lumbodorsal fascia are incised at the lateral border of the quadratus lumborum muscle to reveal the underlying kidney which is invested by Gerota's fascia and surrounded by fat (Fig. 4-5).

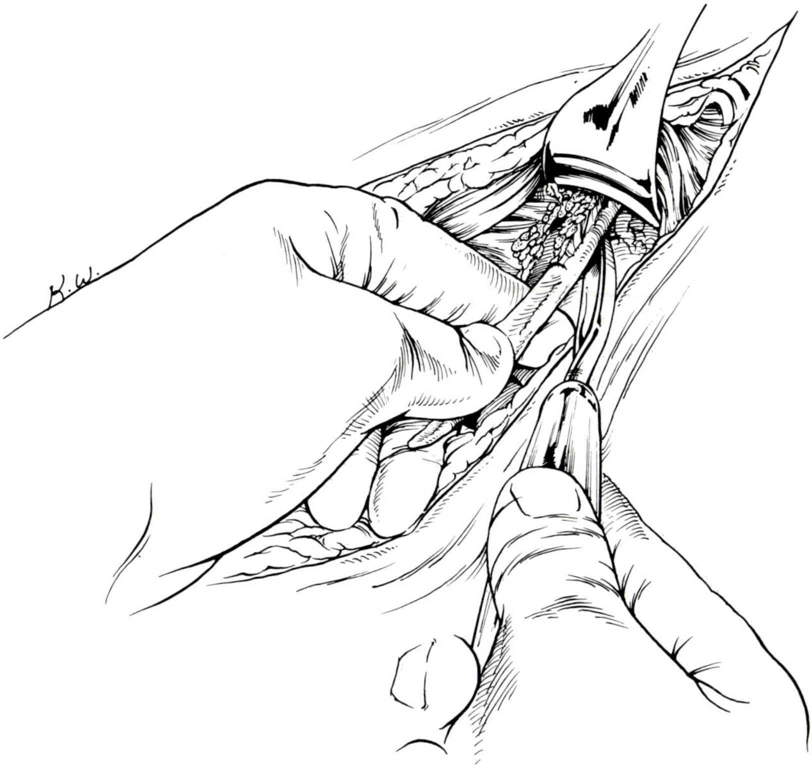

Fig. 4-4. Subperiosteal resection of the right twelfth rib.

Using finger dissection, the fatty and areolar tissues of the suprarenal space are freed up from the undersurface of the diaphragm. Now the diaphragm can be seen as a shelf of muscle with the parietal pleural adherent to its upper surface (Fig. 4-6). The next step is the key to the exposure of the adrenal gland: the pleura is separated from the diaphragm by blunt dissection with a gauze-covered finger and reflected upwards out of the way (Fig. 4-7). The diaphragm can now be divided between large metal clips from its lateral border to the spine without fear of injuring the pleura, to obtain an excellent exposure of the adrenal area (Fig. 4-8).

Gerota's fascia is opened, the kidney is retracted gently downward to bring the adrenal gland prominently into view. The characteristic chrome yellow color of the adrenal gland differs strikingly from that of the surrounding fat and recognition offers no difficulty (Fig. 4-9). The surgeon who is doing this procedure for the first time is usually

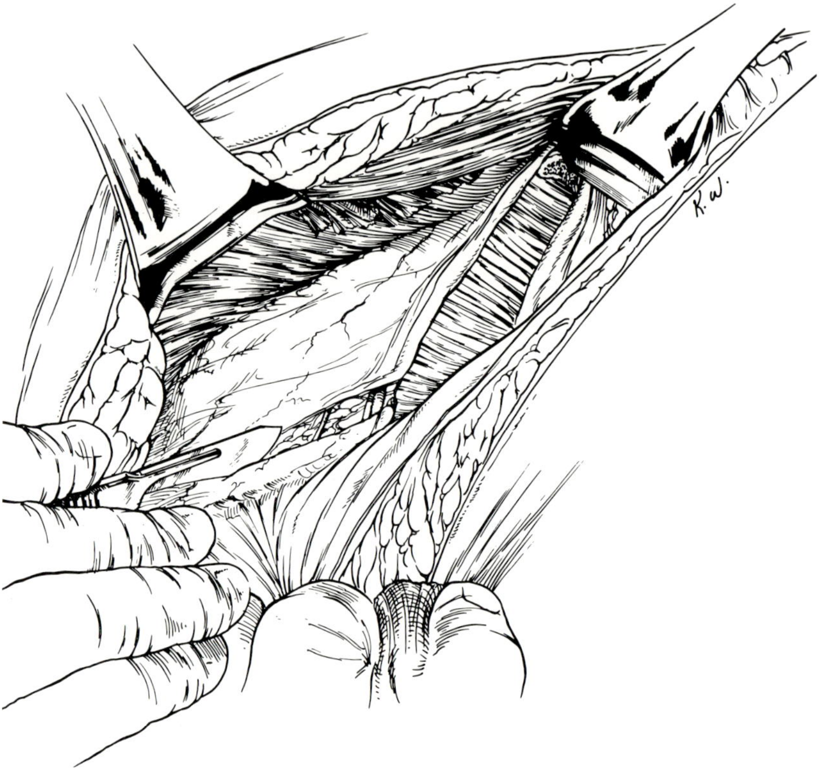

Fig. 4-5. Incision of the right lumbo-dorsal fascia.

surprised to see that the adrenal gland is located more superficially than expected.

The gland is now freed up from its bed proceeding from above downwards. Medium and large tantalum clips (Weck Hemoclips) are used for hemostasis of the many fine vessels which pass between the gland and the surrounding tissues. Each small vessel is individually isolated by gentle dissection with a right-angled clamp. With the vessel supported across the jaws of the clamp a clip is placed on the parietal side and the vessel is divided (Fig. 4-10). There is minimal back bleeding from the adrenal.

The three main adrenal arteries which arise from the aorta and from the phrenic and renal arteries, quickly break up into many fine branches to form a striking arborization around the adrenal. The gland is placed "in the position of a visceral hub of a multispoked vascular wheel."[2] The adrenal veins, on the other hand, have the simplest possible

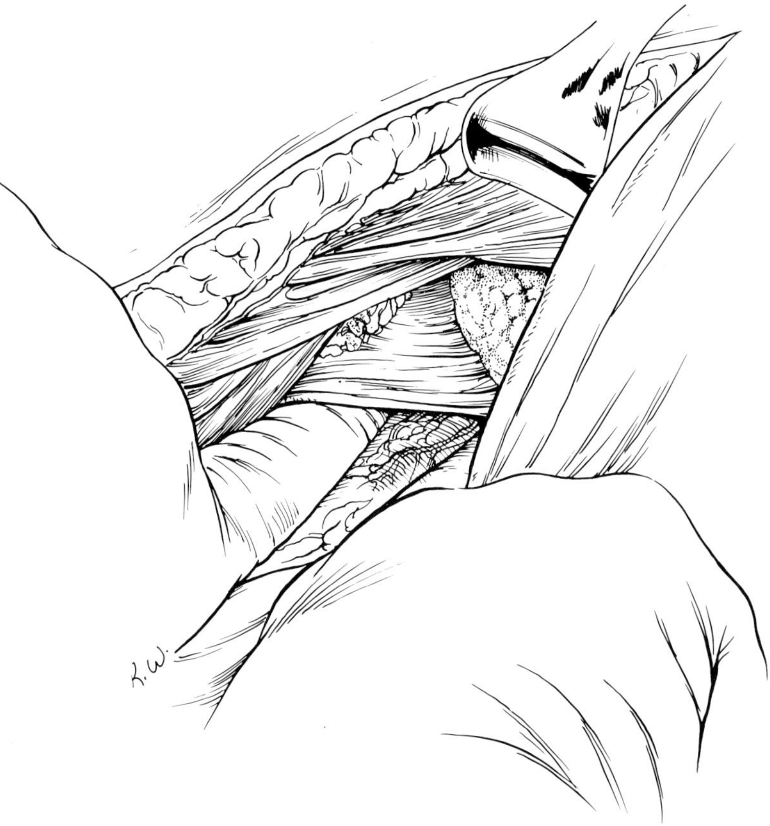

Fig. 4-6. Exposure of the diaphragm by blunt dissection.

arrangement, with one to each gland. The adrenal vein on the right side runs transversely to end abruptly in the inferior vena cava. The left adrenal vein is longer and descends obliquely to enter the left renal vein opposite the gonadal vein. There are very few exceptions to this simple pattern; very occasionally, more than one major vein empties into the vena cava on the right side.

The dissection proceeds methodically until the gland is freed up completely from its bed. The attachments of the gland to the superior pole of the kidney are not divided until the end of the dissection so that the gland will not retract upwards beyond the comfortable reach of the surgeon. Now, only the main venous pedicle remains, it is doubly clipped with large clips—one placed flush with the inferior vena cava or the left renal vein as the case may be, and another just a few mm

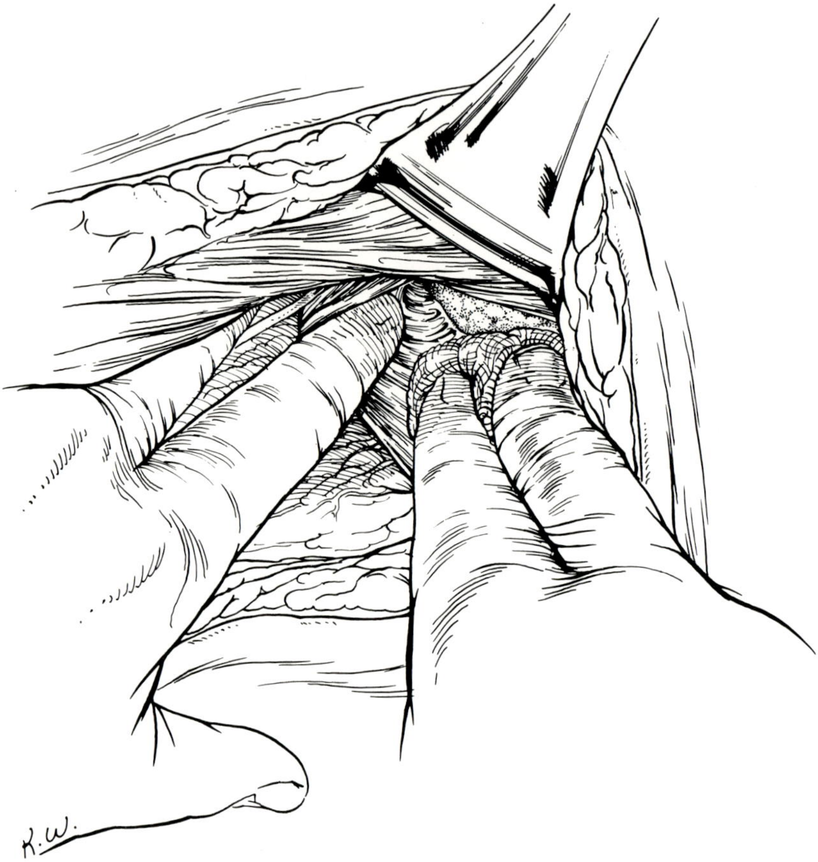

Fig. 4-7. The pleura is reflected superiorly.

distal to it. The vein is divided proximal to the clips and the gland is removed (Fig. 4-11).

Drains are unnecessary, meticulous hemostasis leaves a dry operative field and any dead space is obliterated by perirenal fat. The incision is closed in two layers. The first layer approximates the external edge of the conjoined anterior and middle lamellae of the lumbo-dorsal fascia to the paraspinal muscles (Fig. 4-12). The second layer reunites the edges of the divided posterior lamella of the lumbodorsal fascia. Skin sutures should be left in place for a minimum of 14 days because the incision is subject to unusual stresses and strains due to the stretching and flexing movements of the trunk. This is all the more important in patients who have had adrenalectomy for Cushing's disease; wound healing is significantly retarded in these individuals.

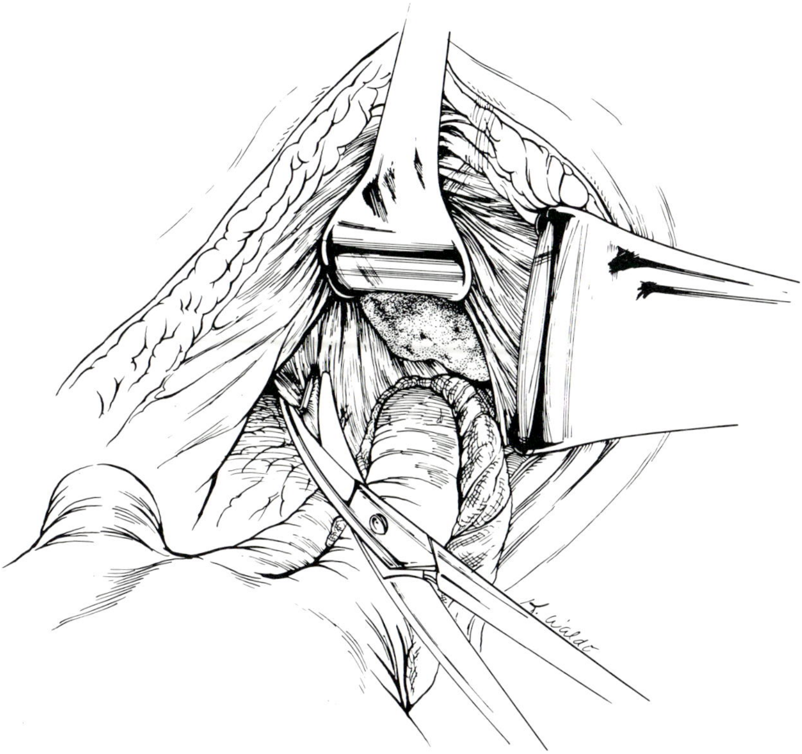

Fig. 4-8. Division of the diaphragm.

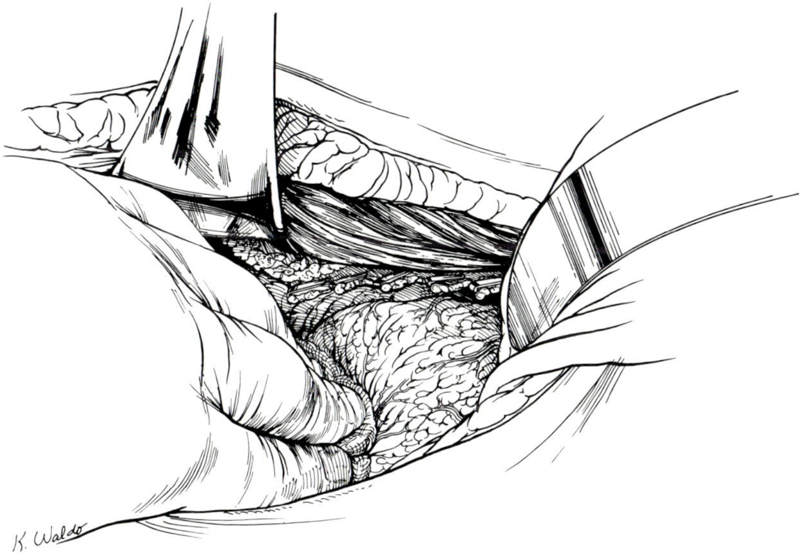

Fig. 4-9. The right adrenal gland is now in view.

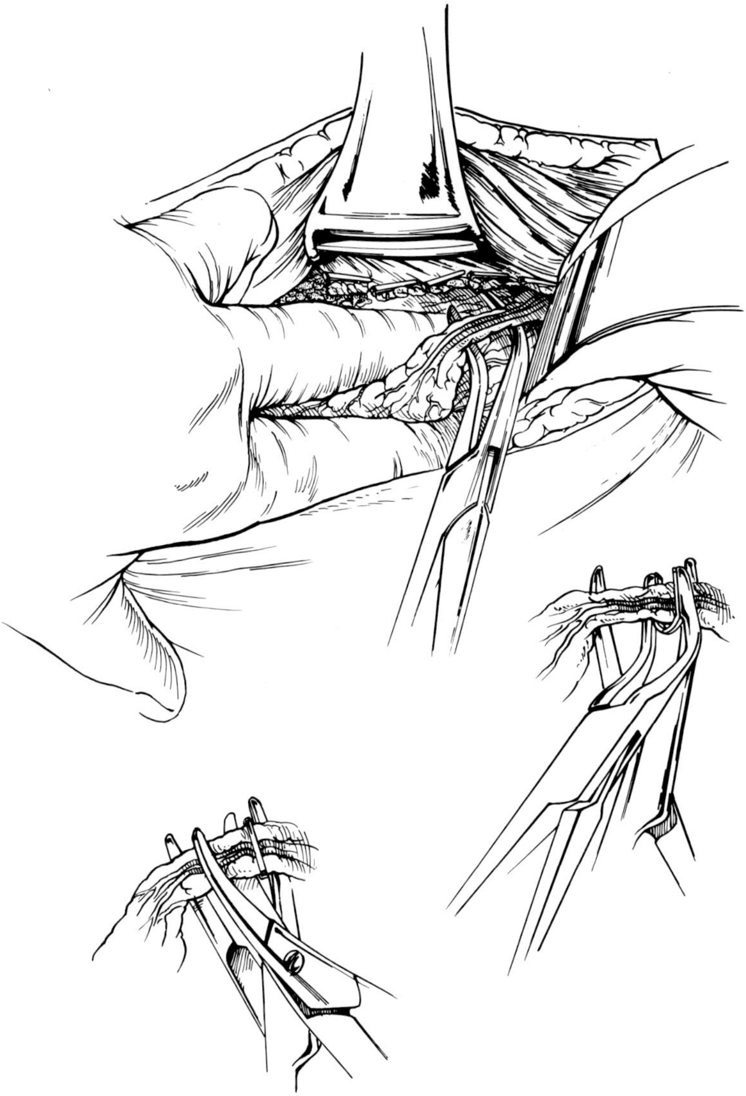

Fig. 4-10. Vessels at the superior aspect of the right adrenal are isolated, clipped and divided.

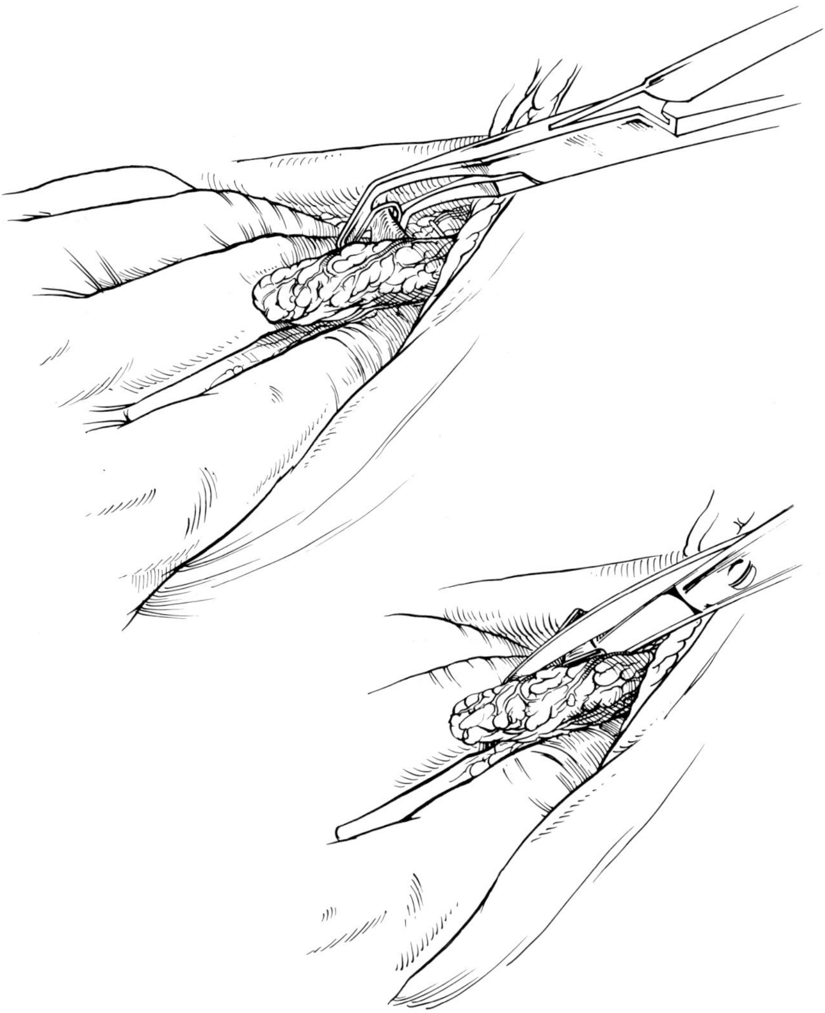

Fig. 4-11. Control of the right adrenal vein at its junction with the inferior vena cava.

Complications

When attention is paid to the technical details outlined above, the incidence of complications can be kept to a minimum.

One of the most serious potential problems is that of bleeding from major venous tears which can occur if the adrenal vein is avulsed by pulling too hard on the gland. This is a rare complication but one should

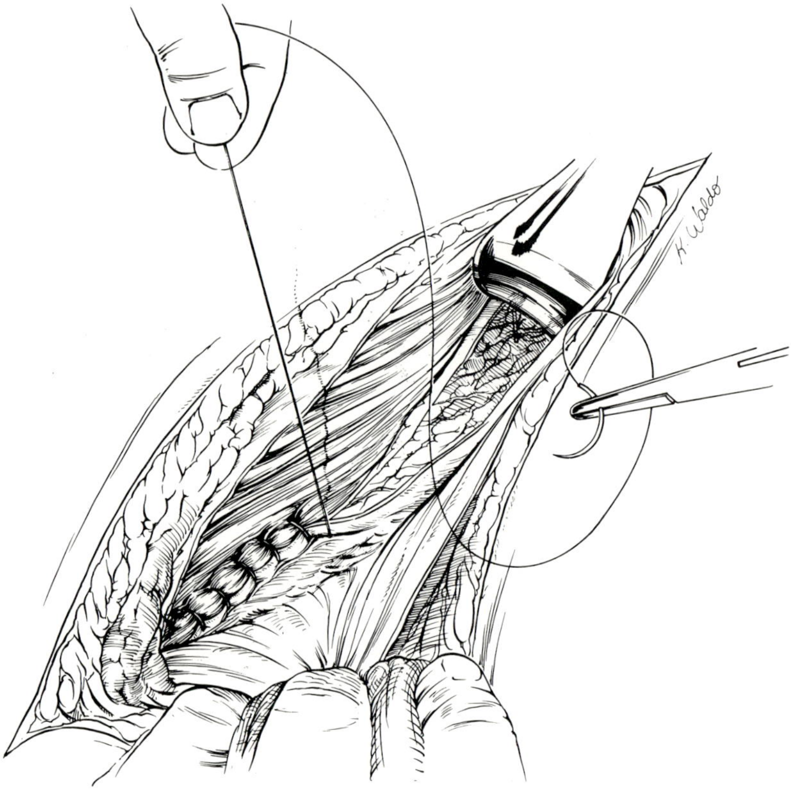

Fig. 4-12. Wound closure. Some surgeons prefer interrupted sutures rather than the continuous suture technique shown.

be prepared to deal with it immediately. Vascular instruments, including a side-biting Satinsky clamp and fine vascular suture material should be included in the routine set-up for adrenalectomy.

Postoperative pneumothorax should be avoidable. When the pleura is inadvertantly torn during the course of the operation, it should be opened widely, and a red rubber catheter inserted into the suprarenal space at the time of wound closure (it isn't necessary to place the tip of the catheter in the actual pleural cavity) and the musculofascial layers are approximated around it. Just prior to closure of the skin, the anesthesiologist overinflates the lungs to empty all the air from the chest via the catheter. With the lungs inflated the catheter is quickly withdrawn. A postoperative chest x-ray is always taken. Should this disclose a significant residual pneumothorax, the air is most conveniently aspirated using a needle, 3-way stopcock and syringe.

Patients have surprisingly little postoperative distress. They complain of less pain than the usual abdominal case, and most are able to move about and cough with comparative ease the day after surgery. The incidence of postoperative pneumonitis and atelectasis is very low.

Because there has been no manipulation of intraperitoneal viscera prolonged postoperative paralytic ileus is most unusual. Pancreatic and splenic injuries are uncommon when the posterior approach to adrenalectomy is used.[6]

When bilateral adrenalectomy is to be performed, 50 mg of hydrocortisone phosphate (cortisol) is given on call to the operating room an intravenous infusion of cortisol at 15 mg per hour is begun with the initial dissection of the adrenals, and continued post-operatively, at a rate of 10 mg per hour for 24 hours. As an additional safety precaution, 50 mg of cortisol is also given intramuscularly every 8 hours so that if the intravenous line infiltrates during the night and is undetected, the patient will still receive an adequate dose of replacement steroid.

After the second postoperative day, the dose of intramuscular cortisol is reduced to 50 mg every 12 hours. On the fifth day, the dose is tapered again, 30 mg being given at 7:00 a.m. and 20 mg at 4:00 p.m. One week postoperatively the intramuscular schedule is changed to the oral route.

Patients with metastatic carcinoma of the breast will usually need a maintenance dose of 50 mg of cortisol per day. Interestingly enough, it is rare to see Cushingoid features develop at this dose. This dose of cortisol will usually provide sufficient mineralocorticoid activity so that special supplementation will not be required. If, however, the maintenance dose of cortisol is decreased below this level, a small dose of synthetic mineralocorticoid (0.05 mg–0.1 mg fluorohydrocortisone) will be required to control sodium metabolism.

If the steroid dose is tapered too rapidly nausea, weakness, fever, depression, and eventually, hypotension will occur. This tendency should be recognized at an early stage and appropriate increments of cortisol given to correct the situation. To avoid fluid retention and water intoxication, in the face of reduced renal free water clearance, intravenous replacement in the early postoperative phase should always be as obligated water, that is as saline (with or without dextrose) and not simply as dextrose and water.

THE ANTERIOR APPROACH TO THE ADRENAL GLAND FOR ADRENAL CORTICAL LESIONS

Satisfactory exploration of the adrenal glands by the anterior approach depends critically upon exposure. Visualization of the adrenals, particularly the right adrenal, is best facilitated by producing exaggerated lordosis. This is generally achieved by elevating a kidney rest beneath the ninth rib. In addition, we use the reverse Trendelenberg position to render the kidneys dependent. The abdomen is opened through a midline incision. Exposure of the right adrenal is achieved by first performing a Kocher maneuver to expose the vena cava. Gerota's fascia is opened and the kidney retracted inferiorly. The vena cava is rotated medially by the first assistant. This permits ultimate exposure of the adrenal vein. The arterial branches to the adrenal are divided after ligation using tantalum clips on the parietal side and long silk ligatures on the adrenal side. These ligatures are left long and provide a convenient means of applying traction to the gland by traction on its vascular stroma. The gland is otherwise too friable to permit traction. When only the medial portion of the dissection remains, the adrenal vein is exposed by lateral traction on the gland and medial rotation of the vena cava. A second adrenal vein entering the vena cava from the superior portion of the adrenal gland is a common feature and requires care. Secure ligation of the adrenal vein or veins is critical to prevent postoperative hemorrhage.

The left adrenal gland is exposed by reflection of the left colon and splenic flexure in the usual manner. Care must be taken to protect the spleen from injury. The tail of the pancreas in retracted superiorly to reveal the left adrenal gland, which is then exposed by opening Gerota's fascia. It is then a simple matter to divide the adrenal vein between ligatures and to dissect the remainder of the gland as in the case of the right adrenal.

The use of tantalum clips expedites the procedure greatly. The abdominal wall is closed with a single layer of interrupted figure of 8 sutures of No. 30 wire.

The anterior approach to the adrenal glands is indicated if there is a need for wide dissection as in adrenal cortical carcinoma, if other abdominal exploration is to be carried out or if it has not been possible for technical reasons to localize an adrenal tumor preoperatively. In addition, this approach may be preferable in all but the most obese patients because of the time saved. In general, the anterior approach is faster than the posterior approach unless two teams are used for bilateral adrenalectomy. The major disadvantage is that it is uniformly accompanied by one or two days of postoperative ileus. There is also a greater incidence of atelectasis unless appropriate respiratory therapy is used. With experience, the degree and duration of ileus can be reduced. Furthermore, the anterior approach requires care to avoid injury to the spleen and tail of the pancreas. These hazards are minimal, however, in the hands of a careful surgeon. The principal adantages of the anterior approach include the ease of access and reduced operative time. In addition, it is not necessary to turn the anesthetized patient who may present with severe osteoporosis and thus with a high risk of fracture. Overall the selection of the anterior or posterior approach must become a matter of individual preference for the surgeon. This in turn will be conditioned by his own experience. We have not had a problem with dehiscence even in the presence of severe Cushing's syndrome, and late appearance of a ventral hernia has been rare.

ANTERIOR TRANSABDOMINAL APPROACH TO THE ADRENAL GLANDS FOR PHEOCHROMOCYTOMA

Indications

The anterior transabdominal approach to the adrenal glands is considered by many to be unwise in Cushing's Disease, and by some to be a source of postoperative morbidity in primary aldosteronism. It is the approach of choice in the surgery of pheochromocytoma. It is recognized that the degree of retroperitoneal dissection and the handling of small bowel inherent in transabdominal exploration of the adrenal glands will create a situation in which postoperative ileus, lasting several days, may develop. This is less true of the posterior and flank approaches to the adrenal gland. Hence, one finds the conviction often stated that the exposure of the adrenal glands through an anterior approach is associated with a higher morbidity that is seen with the flank approach.[5]

Herwig has re-explored, for recurrent Cushing's Disease, two patients in whom the anterior transabdominal approach had been used for the initial attempt at total removal of hyperplastic adrenal glands;[4] Recurrence of the signs of Cushing's Disease was confirmed biochemically and adrenal photoscanning with [^{131}I]iodocholesterol showed uptake in a nodule cradled in a medial retrocaval position on the right side. These patients were re-explored through a right sided flank approach and the cortical remnants removed: one weighing 8 gm and the other 5 gm. Sustained resolution of the Cushing's Disease in both patients has followed the excision of these remnants. Such remnants have not been seen in those patients with Cushing's Disease in whom an initial posterior approach was used for total adrenalectomy.

In pheochromocytoma, roughly 10 percent of the lesions are extra-adrenal and it is possible for the tumors to be found anywhere in the sympathetic chain. For these reasons it is advisable to explore both para-aortic sympathetic chains from the diaphragm to the pelvis in all patients. The exploration can be done effectively through no other approach than a suitable anterior wall abdominal incision.

Incisions

The precise abdominal incision used to approach pheochromocytomas should be individualized to the particular circumstances, i.e., tumor locations, size, and configuration of the abdomen, etc. found in a given patient.

A long midline abdominal incision has given excellent exposure in pre-adolescent children who tend to be thin. Children also have a high incidence of lesions ectopic to the adrenal glands. In such patients, one can reach with ease any point in the abdomen through a midline incision.

In adults, we generally orient the incision toward the lesion because we prefer to remove the pheochromocytoma before undertaking exploration of the para-aortic sympathetic chains. If the patient is somewhat obese and the lesion is in either adrenal gland, a long transverse upper abdominal incision gives sufficient access to the involved adrenal and permits convenient exploration of the para-aortic regions as well.

In their approach to pheochromocytoma of the adrenal gland, H. W. Scott and his collaborators[7] have advocated an upper abdominal incision, palpation of the adrenal glands for verification of the location of the tumor and subsequent extension of the abdominal incision into a thoraco-abdominal approach on the involved side. This approach gives splendid exposure of the adrenal on either side and although we have been prepared to use it on several occasions and have used it deliberately in one, we have not found it routinely necessary in our patients with adrenal pheochromocytoma. The division of the diaphragm and costal cartilage required in the thoraco-abdominal approach to the adrenal glands has a small but nevertheless definite morbidity associated with it.

Para-renal pheochromocytoma and those near the urinary bladder are easily removed through incisions directed toward their specific location in the mid-abdomen or pelvis.

Surgical Approach

GENERAL CONSIDERATIONS

We believe it is important that the capsule of pheochromocytomas, benign or malignant, not be fractured in the course of removal because viable cells may implant and grow in the bed of dissection. Also when-

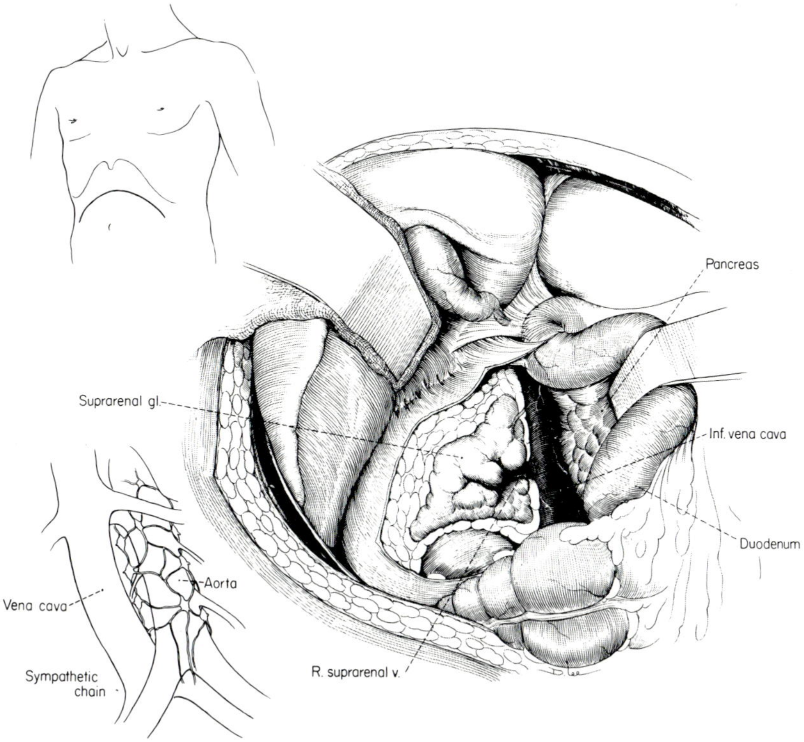

Fig. 4-13. Surgical exposure of the right adrenal gland is shown. The adrenal gland is commonly more superiorly oriented than is apparent in the drawing.

ever it is possible, the major vein draining the pheochromocytoma should be ligated early in the course of dissection.

RIGHT SIDE

With the abdomen opened one should, without delay, expose the involved adrenal gland. On the right side, exposure is usually helped if the hepatic flexure of the colon is widely mobilized and displaced medially and inferiorly (Fig. 4-13). This will expose the retroperitoneal duodenum on the right and, if necessary, the duodenum is also displaced medially after lateral mobilization of the duodenum by a conventional Kocher maneuver.

The right kidney can now be palpated easily and the anterior and right lateral aspect of the inferior vena cava generally comes into plain view. If one gently and sharply explores the space bounded by the superior aspect of the right kidney inferiorly, the vena cava medially and the inferior edge of the posterior aspect of the liver superiorly, the adrenal gland soon will be easily palpated and exposed.

After the right adrenal gland is located, we prefer to develop its lateral and superior aspects early in the dissection. This accomplishes two things; it tends to displace the gland into its most optimum view and secondly makes it easy to manipulate the gland during mobilization of the medial, para-caval aspect of the adrenal. The venous drainage of the right adrenal and its pheochromocytomas is generally found on the medial-posterior aspect of the gland and can be easily controlled if the gland has first been adequately mobilized.

On occasion control of the venous drainage of the right adrenal can be troublesome particularly because the right adrenal vein tends to be short and empties directly into the vena cava. Two precautions minimize difficulties which might occur; one is adequate initial mobilization of the lateral and superior aspects of the right adrenal and the other is to expose the anterior and right lateral aspect of the vena cava widely enough to permit the application of a nontraumatic partial occlusion vascular clamp to the side of the vena cava if it is necessary.

Often a right adrenal pheochromocytoma will have a projection located in a retrocaval position. When this is the case, accurate dissection and gentle intermittent traction on the vena cava will permit safe dissection of the tumor away from the vena cava. The cleavage plane between the tumor and the vena cava is seldom hard to develop.

One should leave as much normal adrenal gland in situ as possible and any bleeding from this adrenal stump can be easily controlled with gently tied figure of eight sutures of fine silk or some other nonabsorbable material.

LEFT SIDE

There are two variations of the transabdominal approach that have been advocated for the left adrenal gland. Both involve division of the gastrocolic ligament on the left side. With the stomach reflected superiorly, the inferior border of the pancreas comes into view (Fig. 4-14). This is mobilized from its inferior aspect and is displaced superiorly along with the stomach. In so doing one encounters the left renal vein and the left adrenal gland, usually with surprising ease. With this approach it is generally a simple matter to expose and ligate the left adrenal vein as it joins the left renal vein. The only important variation on this approach is that frequently it is helpful to widely mobilize the splenic flexure of the colon and this can be most efficiently done as a continuation of the original opening of the gastrocolic omentum.

Particular emphasis should be made on identifying and retracting

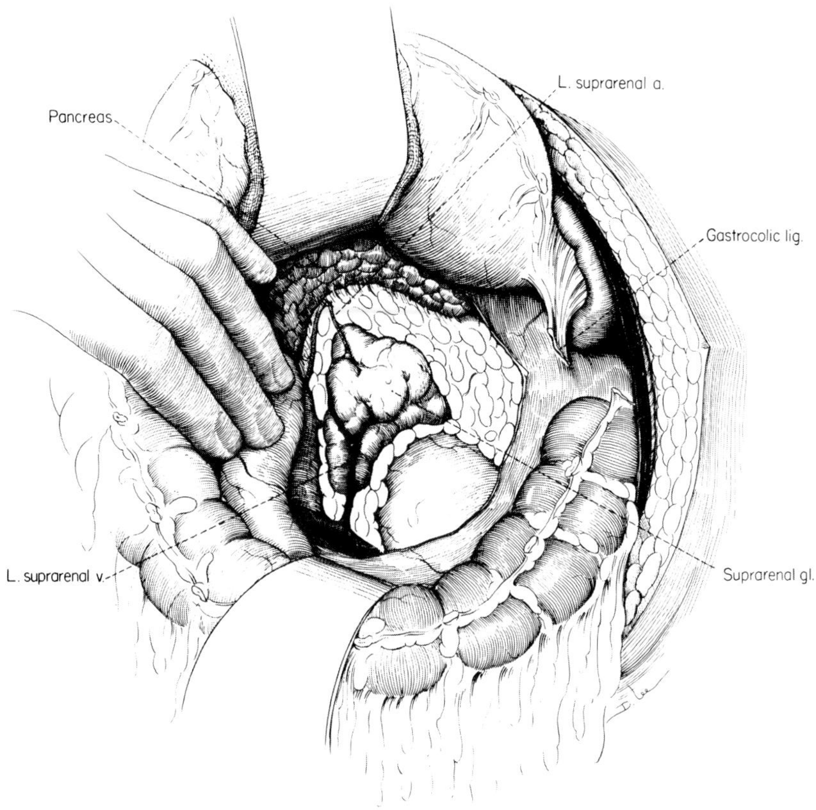

Fig. 4-14. Transabdominal exposure of the left adrenal gland. Unlabelled is the left renal vein into which the left adrenal vein empties. The arterial supply to the gland is seldom as discrete as depicted.

the tail of the pancreas out of harm's way. The tail of the pancreas lies close to the left adrenal, resembles it in consistency and width and can be especially misleading in secondary dissections of the left adrenal.

We have not hesitated to remove the spleen if the exposure of the left adrenal would be cumbersome or difficult without doing so. Splenectomy was a great help with a large cystic left adrenal pheochromocytoma.

EXPLORATION OF THE PARA-AORTIC SYMPATHETIC CHAIN

Every patient with pheochomocytoma should have exploration of the para-aortic sympathetic nerve chain performed at the time of the initial abdominal exploration. To do so does not add a great deal to the operative time and it will exclude the presence of multiple ectopic tumors in the abdomen.

We find it convenient to longitudinally divide the posterior peritoneum overlying the aorta to a point superior to the renal vessels and inferiorly to the bifurcation of the common iliac arteries and urinary bladder.

The sympathetic chains are easily located in their para-aortic positions and their ganglia are frequently a convenient guide in their identification. Particular attention should be paid to the aorto-caval groove on the right side as well as to the retro-caval tissues. On the six occasions we have explored patients for ectopically located macroscopic abdominal pheochromocytoma, it has not been difficult to palpate and remove the lesions in question. One microscopic retro-peritoneal recurrence was found in close proximity to the left lumbar sympathetic chain near the left renal hilum.

REFERENCES

1. Aird I, Helman P: Bilateral anterior transabdominal adrenalectomy. Brit Med J 2:708, 1955
2. Anson BJ, Cauldwell EW, Pick JW, Beaton LE: The blood supply of the kidney, suprarenal gland, and associated structures. Surg. Gym. Obst. 84:313, 1947
3. Crile G: Denervation of the adrenal glands for neurocirculatory asthenia. Surg. Gyn. Obst. 54:294, 1932
4. Herwig KR: Successful removal of adrenal remnant localized by ^{131}I-19-iodocholesterol. J. Urol. 3:713, 1974
5. Nash AG, Robbins GF: The operative approach to the left adrenal gland. Surg. Gyn. Obst. 137:670, 1973
6. Pezzulich RA, Mannix H: Immediate complications of adrenal surgery. Ann Surg 172:125, 1970
7. Scott HW, Riddell DH, Brockman SR: Surgical management of pheochromocytoma. Surg. Gyn. Obst. 120:707, 1965
8. Smithwick RH: Original communications: A technique for splanchnic resection for hypertension. Surgery 7:1, 1940
9. Young HH: A technique for simultaneous exposure and operation on the adrenals. Surg. Gyn. Obst. 54:179, 1936

Index

a b c d e f g h i j
5 6 7 8 9 0 1 2
8